FOREWORD

by *Melissa Castaneda*

I0472506

Being diagnosed with an incurable illness that affects every system of your body is not the life I thought I would be learning in my thirties.
It's also not the life any parent wishes for their children, much less both of their children. My sister also had a lifelong cardiovascular disorder, and I suspect she also had Ehlers-Danlos, but I'm quite positive my mother did not envision this as the ideal future for her children either. Dealing with my own struggles with doctors, specialists and the stress of keeping information organized, feeling dismissed and misunderstood ultimately sparked the idea for this project.
Naturally, knowing the void this journal would fill for the chronic illness community, I began my journey creating and designing the content for you here.

So thank you to my mom for being an avid calendar user her whole life, it fueled the platform for this journal. I hope this creates a communication platform for the chronic illness community that helps to streamline individualized health care and treatment. I am also grateful to have an opportunity to come into your life and help organize your symptoms in ways intended to create more effective therapies, and more importantly a better quality of life.

I would like to dedicate this book to my nieces
Alyssa, Isabella, Jessica, Sophia, Liliana, and Natalia.
Should life present you with seemingly insurmountable situations, just remember you can do and be anything.

Thank you to my family, for putting up with late nights, and going over these layouts over and over!

To the doctors that are genuinely interested in the care of the difficult to treat and extended communities of zebras, your support and understanding means the world to the chronically ill. Please keep doing what you're doing, even if you don't hear 'thank you' as often as you should.
You are appreciated.

To those of us who encounter doctors who have had other interests and provided less than stellar care, do your best to move forward. We are all human, and just because our relationships don't work out the way we envisioned, our tribulations set us up for others who are prepared for us. It's okay to have failures in healthcare, as long as you do not let it prevent you from advocating for yourself and getting the care and treatments you deserve. The journeys can be difficult, but they can also lead to amazing realizations and care.

20 __

to

20 __

Name:

_____

Current Diagnosis:

_____

_____

_____

"The role of the musculoskeletal specialist (e.g., orthopedic surgeon, physiatrist, rehabilitation medicine specialist, rheumatologist) in the care of EDS patients is to help determine the cause of the patient's complaints, and recommend treatment, based on the specific musculoskeletal diagnosis or diagnoses. It is extremely important for the physician to understand the context in which the joint problem occurs, and that the physician understands the individual patient's specific needs and expectations. This requires a thorough understanding of the bodily manifestations of EDS as well as extensive knowledge of the pathophysiology other painful conditions that cause similar symptoms, and appreciating how these problems are affecting the individual person being treated."

-

Ericson Jr WB, Wolman R. 2017. Orthopaedic management of the Ehlers-Danlos Syndromes. Am J Med Genet Part C Semin Med Genet 9999C:1-7

Just as we hold our physicians and caregivers to high standards, we also have a responsibility as patients to provide the most accurate information and accounts of our symptoms, so that we may work together as a team.

EDS Needs, 2018
Circle Where it Hurts©

All rights reserved. Except for the use in reviews, the reproduction or utilization of this work in any form or by any electronic, mechanical, or other means, now known or hereafter invented, including xerography, photocopying, and recording, and in any information storage and retrieval system, is forbidden without the written permission of the publisher.

The web address referenced in this text were current as of April 2018, unless otherwise noted.

- Copyright © 2018 by EDSNeeds
- All rights reserved.
- ISBN-10: 1545175322
- ISBN-13: 978-1545175323

CONTACTS

MEDICAL

PERSONAL

ALLERGIES

〉
〉
〉
〉

THANK YOU!

I would like to take a moment to thank you for your interest in this journal, and commend you on your path to a healthier you. Just setting aside a few moments a day is a gentle way to take reprieve from any stress and just be. Circle Where it Hurts is a collaborative effort to provide information that is lacking in the chronic illness field, namely the Ehlers-Danlos Syndromes. I hope that these volumes of information will provide a much-needed bridge of communication for patients and their caregivers.

For the remainder of this publication I will refer to any person, or persons, acting as your physician, specialists, naturalist, herbalist, or any other licensed caregiver as just that, a caregiver.

Living with any chronic illness is a full-time job and requires constant attention and management by both patients and caregivers. The point of this journal is to provide a chronicle of pertinent and personal information to help you and your caregiver(s) create a tailored plan of action to manage your specific needs.

The idea is to capture all of the inter-related symptoms which occur when you have a syndrome, or any illness, that presents itself with multi-systemic complications and varying comorbidities. The overlapping symptoms, and systems create a virtual tornado of possibilities which can make tailoring a productive and effective method of treatment extremely challenging for caregivers. This journal is intended to create an uninhibited space where you can dialogue with your caregivers so they can step into your pain through the organized compendium of information that you are providing.

No one knows your pain any more clearly than you do, and we cannot expect anyone to fully understand if we are holding back, and even forgetting, important details that can potentially be the key element to productive communication and healing. These journals will reveal the way your pain affects you on a daily bases.

WHAT THIS IS

An open-style journal, designed to assist in the interpretation of complex symptoms. Inside you will find tools, information, and instructions on how to use this journal to its fullest potential.

It was created this way so that it can meet your immediate needs and be used effectively, only purchasing a new journal when you have completed your current one, and not just because the year ran out.

There are several sections dedicated to organize your personal medical information, symptoms, and personal concerns. These sections will focus on identifying symptoms, and your overall health and concerns, so that you can better present your specific medical needs and concerns to your caregiver(s).

HOW I GOT HERE

Pain can manifest itself in so many forms, and translating the information and how deeply it affects you on a daily basis can get lost in translation between the rush to divulge your entire medical history in your allotted 15 minutes of face time with your caregiver and the distractions of life in general. Most importantly the interpretation of your symptoms through tracking, journaling your abnormalities can be a powerful tool of interpretation for your caregivers as to the true root of your pain. Being prepared gives you the opportunity to eliminate otherwise ineffective care, and the frustrations and anxieties that come along with it while you continue to endure your symptoms. This journal intends to create effective communication. Your caregiver can go directly to the information they need to properly create a personalized treatment plan. While this publication is outlined for those with the Ehlers-Danlos Syndromes, the multi-systemic involvement of this condition makes the information, and setup easily adaptable for those with other syndromes/disorders requiring monitoring. If your caregiver is willing to take a few moments to even suggest specifics for you to track, this will help streamline follow-ups. This is why the sections are customizable to fit anyone's needs. If this fits your needs, but you are not a part of the EDS family, please feel free to customize it!

HOW TO USE IT

You will find detailed diagrams in the upcoming pages on how to use the journal section by section. Every patient, illness, and their symptoms are vastly unique. There are several ways you, and your caregivers can customize sections throughout this journal to better fit your needs. Each month will start off with a blank calendar, an overview of your medications, and a free space for you to note any important reminders, or events in the current month. You will also find weekly journal-style content for you to fill with activity, diet, and daily symptoms. This content can also be used as indicated or customized to your illness, or symptom requirements. As you begin to complete monthly entries, paper clipping, or separating the months in any way will create a more cohesive presentation for anyone to navigate.

WHY

Because the Ehlers-Danlos Syndromes are highly under-researched and misunderstood. Because those suffering deserve a clear voice. Because after the flare ups, and chronic pain, it's easy to forget what you wanted to go over with your caregiver, and waiting months to reschedule with any specialists only catalyzes anxiety and depression, which can compromise your already overly stressed systems.
There has to be a better way to communicate.
Let this journal be your voice.

OVERVIEW

- The Ehlers-Danlos syndromes are a group of heritable connective tissue disorders. It is multisystemic, and can affect every patient differently.
- EDS can range from benign symptoms, to life-threatening complications.
- This journal is in no way intended to serve as diagnostic criteria, or replace therapies, medications, or the advice from your caregiver.
- Always consult your caregiver if you have any new symptoms, concerns, or questions.
- Ehlers Danlos can be, and is largely, and invisible condition.
- The Ehlers-Danlos syndromes are known to present themselves with complications in the following systems:

CARDIOVASCULAR
GASTROINTESTINAL
ORTHOPAEDIC
NEUROLOGICAL AND SPINAL
ORAL AND MANDIBULAR
SYCHOLOGICAL AND PSYCHIATRIC
CELLULAR
IMPAIRMENT OF THE PROPRIOCEPTIVE SENSE

- Accuracy and honesty are paramount when journaling your symptoms, for your best treatment options.

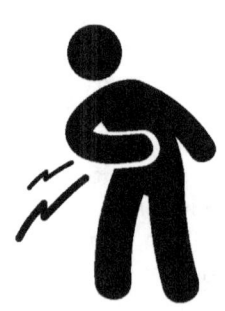

CARDIOVASCULAR

- Orthostatic Intolerance - OI
- Orthostatic Hypotension - OH
- Neurally Mediated Hypotension - NMH
- Postural Tachycardia Syndrome - POTS
- Low blood pressure
- Increased venous dilation and blood pooling
- low circulating blood volume

GASTROINTESTINAL

- Chronic Constipation/diarrhea
- Uterine/Rectal Prolapse
- GI Bleeding
- Motility Issues
- Small Bowel Dysmotility
- Delayed Gastric Emptying
- Delayed Colonic Transit

ORTHOPAEDIC

- Joint hypermobility
- Acute and chronic pain
- Cervical Spine Instability
- Shoulder instability
- Hip instability
- Thumb instability
- Wrist instability
- Lumbar spine instability
- Thoracic Outlet Syndrome
- Elbow instability
- Finger instability
- Knee instability
- Ankle instability
- Foot instability
- Nerve issues due to instability
- Proprioception issues

NEURO/SPINAL

- Headaches
- Migraines
- Chiari I Malformation - CMI
- Idiopathic Intracranial Hypertension - IIH
- Atlantoaxial Instability
- Craniocervical Instability - CCI
- Segmental Kyphosis and Instability
- Tethered Cord Syndrome
- Dystonia
- Movement Disorders
- Neuromuscular pain
- Peripheral Neuropathy
- Nerve Pain

ORAL/MANDIBULAR

- TMJ Hypermobility
- Temporomandibular Dysfunction - TMD

PSYCHIATRIC

- Anxiety
- Depression
- Mood disorders
- Eating disorders
- Neurodevelopmental disorders

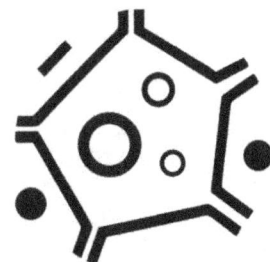

CELLULAR

- Mast Cell Activation Disorder & Syndrome
- skin flushing/pruritis/urticaria/angioedema
- diarrhea/bloating/cramping
- rhinitis
- anaphylaxis/stinging insect allergy/
- peri-operative anaphylaxis

THE LAYOUT

1. Each monthly section will start with a blank calendar which will reflect the current month. You will need to fill out each calendar at the beginning of each month (preferably).
2. Directly after the calendar month, there will be a Month in Review section where you can record your medications, reactions and pertinent monthly symptoms. Sections 1 and 2 will be displayed in a traditional calendar format to help organize sections and information.
3. This will be followed by your weekly logs where you can record everything from diet, to activity, to daily symptoms, or customize one or more sections for a more personalized experience.
4. At the end of each week you will find a section for notes, and a Week in Motion section which we will go over in greater detail in the following pages.

1

- Fill out the first page of this book with your starting month/year information
- Dating all of the months at once can be daunting. If it's too much at once, you can do this as the months start!
- Refer to the extended yearly calendars at the end of the journal for relative monthly dates.
- You can use index stickers to divide months for easy navigating as your logs begin to fill up.

SEPTEMBER

SUN/DOM	MON/LUN	TUES/MAR	WEDS/MIE	THURS/JUE	FRI/VIE	SAT/SA
					1	2
3	4 HOLIDAY	5	6	7 OPTOMETRY 2:00 P.M.	8 1ST DAY OF SCHOOL PHYSIO 10:30	9
10 SOCCER 5 P.M.	11	12	13 NEURO 9:00 A.M.	14	15	16
17 SOCCER 5 P.M.	18	19	20	21 GASTRO 1:30 P.M.	22 PHYSIO 10:30 A.M.	23
24 SOCCER 5 P.M.	25	26	27	28	29	30

Notes
DAD'S BIRTHDAY NEXT MONTH, 13TH. GET CARD BEFORE THE END OF THE MONTH.

2

MONTH IN REVIEW

Current Meds
- FLUOXETINE - 20 MG/DAILY

Reactions
- DECREASED ANXIETY
- ABDOMINAL PAIN

New Meds
- SUMATRIPTAN - 100 MG/ AS NEEDED

Reactions
- LESSENED MAJOR MIGRAINE WITH AURA, BUT DID NOT COMPLETELY ALLEVIATE

Supplements
- GABACALM
- ARNICA
- TURMERIC
- MATCHA
- MACA
- B12 - CYANOCABALAMIN

Reactions
- NO REACTION
- ACCELERATED BRUISE HEALING
- DECREASED OVERALL JOINT PAIN
- INCREASED ENERGY
- HAIR GROWTH
- NONE YET

NOTES
FELL ON L HIP ON THE 28TH, PERSISTENT PAIN FOR THE FOLLOWING 2 WEEKS. SEE JOURNAL ENTRY FOR SPECIFICS.

Use this space to assess and prioritize pain/severity/persistence/ Location in terms of importance so you don't forget to pass on important information. Walking away from an appointment and realizing you've completely forgotten to go over what you needed to can be beyond frustrating.

WOMEN'S HEALTH

Symptoms/Cycle
- LEFT OVARY SENSITIVITY NOT CORRELATED WITH CYCLE.
- 12-18

EDS is by far more prevalent in women. Irregular cycles are important to log for your caregiver. Menorrhagia, dysmenorrhea, excessive bleeding or pain can be debilitating, and need to be addressed with your caregiver. You can also use this space to record your monthly cycle dates for quick reference.

MEN'S HEALTH

Symptoms
- DIFFICULTY URINATING
- ON THE 12TH 25TH & 31ST

Did you know difficulty urinating, frequent urination, and the inability to urinate are seemingly harmless events, but can be primary indicators of issues with your prostate? Don't forget to record any related symptoms or sensations.

HOW TO USE YOUR LOG

These headings are designed to have you
log specific habits and symptoms so that your
disease/sickness/illness/syndrome can be represented
in context to you and how your specific injuries and symptoms occur.

You can use the logs as they are, using the Legend below throughout your use of this journal.
Or use the space to the right of the abbreviated Legend headings in the daily logs to
personalize your logging needs.

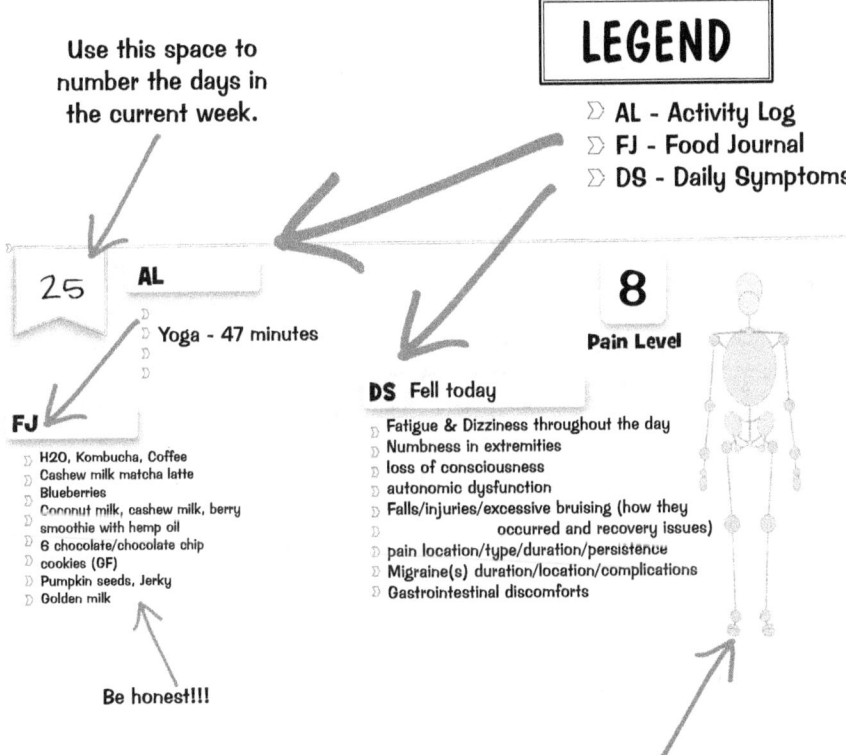

Use this space to
number the days in
the current week.

LEGEND

> AL - Activity Log
> FJ - Food Journal
> DS - Daily Symptoms

25 **AL**

> Yoga - 47 minutes

FJ

> H2O, Kombucha, Coffee
> Cashew milk matcha latte
> Blueberries
> Coconut milk, cashew milk, berry
> smoothie with hemp oil
> 6 chocolate/chocolate chip
> cookies (GF)
> Pumpkin seeds, Jerky
> Golden milk

Be honest!!!

8

Pain Level

DS Fell today

> Fatigue & Dizziness throughout the day
> Numbness in extremities
> loss of consciousness
> autonomic dysfunction
> Falls/injuries/excessive bruising (how they
>   occurred and recovery issues)
> pain location/type/duration/persistence
> Migraine(s) duration/location/complications
> Gastrointestinal discomforts

We'll get to this guy in a moment.

FILLING IN YOUR LOGS

- Do you move for at least five minutes a day? Any activity is good activity!
- You may have become accustomed to nagging pains, but your caregivers are not. Use accurate descriptive words when relaying pain information. A list of words will be listed under the upcoming 'descriptive dialogue' section.
- That burning or shooting pain can be important when diagnosing or navigating a plan of action.
- Write it down, and be specific!
- Food can directly affect and even trigger symptoms. Keeping a food journal is a huge investigative tool for your caregivers.
- Using these spaces to their potential only increases accurate communication.
- No one knows your pain more clearly than you do, help your caregivers help you.

LET'S TALK PAIN

- Did you know that when you are asked to "rate your pain,"
your doctor may be referring to a scale you may be
unfamiliar with. Let's all get on the same page, and rate our
pain according to the following guidelines.
These guidelines are designed to interpret the
Wong Baker Pain Scale in terms of your
ability to perform activities. When you hand this journal to your
provider for the first time, have them review this scale so we're
all speaking the same language. Use this scale to determine your daily Pain
Scale level.

WHAT ARE SOME OF YOUR PAIN TRIGGERS?

> Use the scale below to help identify
> movements, activities and other triggers that
> instigate spikes in pain and alterations of mobility to
> help determine your applicable pain levels.
> This will also help you identify mentionable events in
> your 'month in review' section for caregivers.

Pain Level

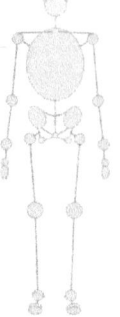

ACTIVITY LEVEL SCALE

0 — Pain free.

Mild Pain — Nagging, annoying, but doesn't really interfere with daily living activities.

1 — Pain is very mild, barely noticeable. Most of the time you don't think about it.

2 — Minor pain. Annoying and may have occasional stronger twinges.

3 — Pain is noticeable and distracting, however, you can get used to it and adapt.

Moderate Pain — Interferes significantly with daily living activities.

4 — Moderate pain. If you are deeply involved in an activity, it can be ignored for a period of time, but is still distracting.

5 — Moderately strong pain. It can't be ignored for more than a few minutes, but with effort you still can manage to work or participate in some social activities.

6 — Moderately strong pain that interferes with normal daily activities. Difficulty concentrating.

Severe Pain — Disabling; unable to perform daily living activities.

7 — Severe pain that dominates your senses and significantly limits your ability to perform normal daily activities or maintain social relationships. Interferes with sleep.

8 — Intense pain. Physical activity is severely limited. Conversing requires great effort

9 — Excruciating pain. Unable to converse. Crying out and/or moaning uncontrollably.

10 — Unspeakable pain. Bedridden and possibly delirious.

MEET YOUR PAIN REP. - ART

This Anatomic Representation Tool, ART, is printed on every daily journal and will represent your symptoms so that your caregiver(s) can visually appreciate how exhausting your daily experiences are. Anything you log in your journals can be represented on ART. You can simply circle each symptomatic area for the day, or create a personalized legend on the next couple of pages representing the types of pain you experience most frequently. For example, different types of neuropathic pain, dizziness, and types of gastrointestinal issues. Also, legends can be useful when trying to identify types of pain when there are several organs present. For example, if you were to circle the lower portion of the abdomen, is it your hip, intestines, bladder, or spine?
You have different organs on different sides of your body as well, so making sure you place your markings on the correct side will be beneficial.

example

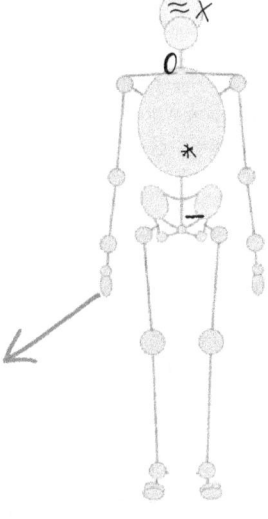

LEGEND

- ▷ X - AUDITORY
- ▷ O - NECK
- ▷ — - UTERINE
- ▷ * - NAUSEA
- ▷ ~ DIZZINESS

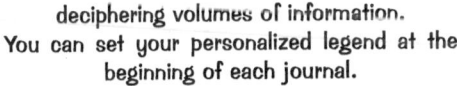

- As you can see by these few examples, if you have chronic shoulder pain, circling too close to the neck area might be confusing.
Using simple markings, or even colored codes, will be monumental in deciphering volumes of information.
You can set your personalized legend at the beginning of each journal.

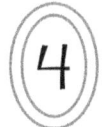

Pain Level

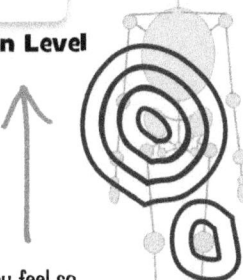

If you feel so inclined, you can average your weekly pain level in this space.

- At the end of each week you will find your "Week in Motion" section. Use this section to brain dump, solve life's mysteries, or just write any important notes. This space has endless possibilities so get creative!

- We've placed an 8th, and optional, pain representative here for a little visual exercise. I encourage you to try this for at least a few months.

- At the end of each week go back through your daily symptoms and for each symptom noted, circle the corresponding location on ART once for that day. If you note pain in that area any other day of the week, create an additional/larger circle around the same area for each day it is noted (no one area should be circled more than 7 times). You will begin to see your pain come alive at the end of the first month or so, and at the end of the year you will have your own flipbook of visual pain.

TIPS

Journaling can seem like a daunting task, but if you can dedicate a few minutes a day to outlining your illness for others you can make this work!

- For quick reference use the contacts section at the beginning of your journal to keep your team of caregivers information handy. You can update information mid-way through the journal in the "6-month check-in" section half way through the workbook.

- Time associations can help create an easy way to remember to sit down with your journal every day. Try always journaling at the same time, or during the same activity every day. This can also be an effective way to incorporate journaling if this a new activity for you. Try thinking of this activity like a "brain dump" so to speak. Once you have logged all of your symptoms and concerns, you can rest with a clean slate ready for the new day. I realize journaling is not always possible, however please try to journal as consistently as possible for the most accurate information. Accuracy and honesty is key!

- If you've discovered any tips that you need to make note of throughout your experience using your journal, please use the space below to jot them down!

- Make it fun. Incorporate colors, stamps, or stickers to help you get into the groove of journaling if you've never tried it before.
- Not a stamper? Log other monthly activities or sports you participate in.

- In addition to the free space throughout your daily entries, there will also be designated pages for notes at the end of each month, should you need to record symptoms, thoughts, or events of importance.

- If you ever get lost, refer back to these examples, check us out online for help, or email in!
  1. edsneeds@gmail.com
  2. www.edsneeds.com

- Use the 6-month check-in section to update any new allergies, intolerances, major diagnostic findings, and update contacts.

TIPS/TRICKS

DESCRIPTIVE DIALOGUE

- Using descriptive dialogue to narrate your symptoms helps caregivers decipher types of pain and their root causes. You can even use some of these for your personalized legend if you see them popping up frequently.
- If you are using this journal for any other illness, please use the blank bulleted fields to enter your own criteria for you to refer to easily.
- These can coordinate to headings in your daily logs that you may have changed.

LOCATION

- Left/Right Arm
- Left/Right Leg
- Left/Right Hand
- Left/Right Shoulder
- Left/Right Jaw
- Left/Right Foot
- Upper/Lower/Mid Back
- Left/Right Head
- Left/Right Eye

DURATION

- Seconds
- Minutes

If you start to see patterns you can use words like

- Days
- Weeks

in the weekly recap section, Week In Motion.

TYPES OF PAIN

- Sharp
- Aching
- Burning
- Stinging
- Dull
- Throbbing
- Squeezing
- Cramping
- Constant
- Shooting
- Numbing
- Crushing
- Pins/Needles

USING YOUR LEGEND

- This will be your legend for the remainder of your journal. Place an index tab here so that you and your caregivers can find this point of reference easily.
- You can also use this space to note any important information regarding specific recurring symptoms.

MY PAIN LEGEND

〉
〉
〉
〉
〉
〉
〉

〉
〉
〉
〉
〉
〉
〉

SUN/DOM	MON/LUN	TUES/MAR	WEDS/MIE	THURS/JUE	FRI/VIE	SAT/SA

Notes

MONTH IN REVIEW

Current Meds
> >
> >
> >
> >

New Meds
> >
> >
> >
> >

Supplements
> >
> >
> >
> >
> >
> >

Reactions
> >
> >
> >
> >

Reactions
> >
> >
> >
> >

Reactions
> >
> >
> >
> >
> >
> >

WOMEN'S HEALTH

Symptoms/Cycle
> >
> >
> >
> >

MEN'S HEALTH

Symptoms
> >
> >
> >
> >

NOTES

QUESTIONS FOR YOUR CAREGIVER

Date/type of appointment:

_____

ANSWERS

Date/type of appointment:

_____

ANSWERS

Date/type of appointment:

_____

ANSWERS

NOTES

BLOOD WORK AND TESTS

Requested by Dr.:
Test for:
Prep:
Result:
Follow-up:

Requested by Dr.:
Test for:
Prep:
Result:
Follow-up:

Requested by Dr.:
Test for:
Prep:
Result:
Follow-up:

Requested by Dr.:
Test for:
Prep:
Result:
Follow-up:

TO-DO

Do something EVERY DAY that inspires you.

SUN/DOM	MON/LUN	TUES/MAR	WEDS/MIE	THURS/JUE	FRI/VIE	SAT/SA

Notes

MONTH IN REVIEW

Current Meds
- ◇
- ◇
- ◇
- ◇

New Meds
- ◇
- ◇
- ◇
- ◇

Supplements
- ◇
- ◇
- ◇
- ◇
- ◇
- ◇

Reactions
- ◇
- ◇
- ◇
- ◇

Reactions
- ◇
- ◇
- ◇
- ◇

Reactions
- ◇
- ◇
- ◇
- ◇
- ◇
- ◇

WOMEN'S HEALTH

Symptoms/Cycle
- ◇
- ◇
- ◇
- ◇

MEN'S HEALTH

Symptoms
- ◇
- ◇
- ◇
- ◇

NOTES

QUESTIONS FOR YOUR CAREGIVER

Date/type of appointment:

_____

ANSWERS

Date/type of appointment:

_____

ANSWERS

Date/type of appointment:

_____

ANSWERS

NOTES

BLOOD WORK AND TESTS

Requested by Dr.:
Test for:
Prep:
Result:
Follow-up:

Requested by Dr.:
Test for:
Prep:
Result:
Follow-up:

Requested by Dr.:
Test for:
Prep:
Result:
Follow-up:

Requested by Dr.:
Test for:
Prep:
Result:
Follow-up:

TO-DO

Don't ever save anything for a special occasion.
Being alive is the special occasion. – UNK

SUN/DOM	MON/LUN	TUES/MAR	WEDS/MIE	THURS/JUE	FRI/VIE	SAT/SA

Notes

MONTH IN REVIEW

Current Meds
- ☆
- ☆
- ☆
- ☆

Reactions
- ☆
- ☆
- ☆
- ☆

New Meds
- ☆
- ☆
- ☆
- ☆

Reactions
- ☆
- ☆
- ☆
- ☆

Supplements
- ☆
- ☆
- ☆
- ☆
- ☆
- ☆

Reactions
- ☆
- ☆
- ☆
- ☆
- ☆
- ☆

NOTES

WOMEN'S HEALTH

Symptoms/Cycle
- ☆
- ☆
- ☆
- ☆

MEN'S HEALTH

Symptoms
- ☆
- ☆
- ☆
- ☆

QUESTIONS FOR YOUR CAREGIVER

Date/type of appointment:

_____

ANSWERS

Date/type of appointment:

_____

ANSWERS

Date/type of appointment:

_____

ANSWERS

NOTES

BLOOD WORK AND TESTS

Requested by Dr.:
Test for:
Prep:
Result:
Follow-up:

Requested by Dr.:
Test for:
Prep:
Result:
Follow-up:

Requested by Dr.:
Test for:
Prep:
Result:
Follow-up:

Requested by Dr.:
Test for:
Prep:
Result:
Follow-up:

TO-DO

Do the thing you fear the most and the death of fear is certain.

– Mark Twain

SUN/DOM	MON/LUN	TUES/MAR	WEDS/MIE	THURS/JUE	FRI/VIE	SAT/SA

Notes

MONTH IN REVIEW

Current Meds

◇ ◇ ◇ ◇ ◇

New Meds

◇ ◇ ◇ ◇ ◇

Supplements

◇ ◇ ◇ ◇ ◇ ◇ ◇

Reactions

◇ ◇ ◇ ◇ ◇

Reactions

◇ ◇ ◇ ◇ ◇

Reactions

◇ ◇ ◇ ◇ ◇ ◇

NOTES

WOMEN'S HEALTH

Symptoms/Cycle

◇ ◇ ◇ ◇

MEN'S HEALTH

Symptoms

◇ ◇ ◇ ◇

QUESTIONS FOR YOUR CAREGIVER

Date/type of appointment:

_____

ANSWERS

Date/type of appointment:

_____

ANSWERS

Date/type of appointment:

_____

ANSWERS

NOTES

BLOOD WORK AND TESTS

Requested by Dr.:
Test for:
Prep:
Result:
Follow-up:

Requested by Dr.:
Test for:
Prep:
Result:
Follow-up:

Requested by Dr.:
Test for:
Prep:
Result:
Follow-up:

Requested by Dr.:
Test for:
Prep:
Result:
Follow-up:

TO-DO

Self Care IS Health Care.

SUN/DOM	MON/LUN	TUES/MAR	WEDS/MIE	THURS/JUE	FRI/VIE	SAT/SA

Notes

MONTH IN REVIEW

Current Meds

⌐ ⌐ ⌐ ⌐
⌐ ⌐ ⌐ ⌐
⌐ ⌐

New Meds

⌐ ⌐ ⌐ ⌐
⌐ ⌐ ⌐ ⌐

Supplements

⌐ ⌐ ⌐ ⌐
⌐ ⌐ ⌐ ⌐
⌐ ⌐ ⌐

Reactions

⌐ ⌐ ⌐
⌐ ⌐ ⌐
⌐ ⌐

Reactions

⌐ ⌐ ⌐
⌐ ⌐ ⌐

Reactions

⌐ ⌐ ⌐
⌐ ⌐ ⌐
⌐ ⌐

NOTES

WOMEN'S HEALTH

Symptoms/Cycle

⌐ ⌐ ⌐
⌐ ⌐

MEN'S HEALTH

Symptoms

⌐ ⌐ ⌐
⌐ ⌐

QUESTIONS FOR YOUR CAREGIVER

Date/type of appointment:

_____

ANSWERS

Date/type of appointment:

_____

ANSWERS

Date/type of appointment:

_____

ANSWERS

NOTES

BLOOD WORK AND TESTS

Requested by Dr.:
Test for:
Prep:
Result:
Follow-up:

Requested by Dr.:
Test for:
Prep:
Result:
Follow-up:

Requested by Dr.:
Test for:
Prep:
Result:
Follow-up:

Requested by Dr.:
Test for:
Prep:
Result:
Follow-up:

TO-DO

You ARE worth it.

SUN/DOM	MON/LUN	TUES/MAR	WEDS/MIE	THURS/JUE	FRI/VIE	SAT/SA	

Notes

MONTH IN REVIEW

Current Meds
☆ ☆ ☆ ☆

Reactions
☆ ☆ ☆ ☆

New Meds
☆ ☆ ☆ ☆

Reactions
☆ ☆ ☆ ☆

Supplements
☆ ☆ ☆ ☆ ☆ ☆

Reactions
☆ ☆ ☆ ☆ ☆

NOTES

WOMEN'S HEALTH

Symptoms/Cycle
☆ ☆ ☆ ☆

MEN'S HEALTH

Symptoms
☆ ☆ ☆ ☆

QUESTIONS FOR YOUR CAREGIVER

Date/type of appointment:

_____

ANSWERS

Date/type of appointment:

_____

ANSWERS

Date/type of appointment:

_____

ANSWERS

NOTES

BLOOD WORK AND TESTS

Requested by Dr.:
Test for:
Prep:
Result:
Follow-up:

Requested by Dr.:
Test for:
Prep:
Result:
Follow-up:

Requested by Dr.:
Test for:
Prep:
Result:
Follow-up:

Requested by Dr.:
Test for:
Prep:
Result:
Follow-up:

TO-DO

What if I fall? Oh but my darling, what if you FLY?
- ERIN HANSON

6-MONTH CHECK-IN

- Use this space to log important diagnostic findings and update important medical information like new allergies.
- Please make sure you note life-saving instructions should caregivers and loved ones forget out of fear and confusion during an emergency situation.
- An additional contact sheet has been added to accommodate for new and/or changing specialists.

UPDATED MEDICAL INFORMATION

ALLERGIES

TEST RESULTS

Don't forget to date and label test results.

YOU'RE SIX MONTHS INTO LOGGING, *congratulations!*
IF YOU'VE BEEN CONTRIBUTING TO YOUR WEEK IN MOTION FIGURES,
TAKE A MOMENT TO FLIP THROUGH THE LAST SIX MONTHS AND
WATCH YOUR PROGRESSION OF PAIN.

MEDICAL

PERSONAL

SUN/DOM	MON/LUN	TUES/MAR	WEDS/MIE	THURS/JUE	FRI/VIE	SAT/SA

Notes

MONTH IN REVIEW

Current Meds
- ⌂
- ⌂
- ⌂
- ⌂

New Meds
- ⌂
- ⌂
- ⌂
- ⌂

Supplements
- ⌂
- ⌂
- ⌂
- ⌂
- ⌂
- ⌂

Reactions
- ⌂
- ⌂
- ⌂
- ⌂

Reactions
- ⌂
- ⌂
- ⌂
- ⌂

Reactions
- ⌂
- ⌂
- ⌂
- ⌂
- ⌂
- ⌂

NOTES

WOMEN'S HEALTH

Symptoms/Cycle
- ⌂
- ⌂
- ⌂
- ⌂

MEN'S HEALTH

Symptoms
- ⌂
- ⌂
- ⌂
- ⌂

QUESTIONS FOR YOUR CAREGIVER

Date/type of appointment:

_____

ANSWERS

Date/type of appointment:

_____

ANSWERS

Date/type of appointment:

_____

ANSWERS

NOTES

BLOOD WORK AND TESTS

Requested by Dr.:
Test for:
Prep:
Result:
Follow-up:

Requested by Dr.:
Test for:
Prep:
Result:
Follow-up:

Requested by Dr.:
Test for:
Prep:
Result:
Follow-up:

Requested by Dr.:
Test for:
Prep:
Result:
Follow-up:

TO-DO

Life is better when you're laughing – UNK

SUN/DOM	MON/LUN	TUES/MAR	WEDS/MIE	THURS/JUE	FRI/VIE	SAT/SA

Notes

MONTH IN REVIEW

Current Meds

☆ ☆ ☆ ☆ ☆

New Meds

☆ ☆ ☆ ☆ ☆

Supplements

☆ ☆ ☆ ☆ ☆ ☆

Reactions

☆ ☆ ☆ ☆ ☆

Reactions

☆ ☆ ☆ ☆ ☆

Reactions

☆ ☆ ☆ ☆ ☆

NOTES

WOMEN'S HEALTH

Symptoms/Cycle

☆ ☆ ☆ ☆

MEN'S HEALTH

Symptoms

☆ ☆ ☆ ☆

QUESTIONS FOR YOUR CAREGIVER

Date/type of appointment:

_____

ANSWERS

Date/type of appointment:

_____

ANSWERS

Date/type of appointment:

_____

ANSWERS

NOTES

BLOOD WORK AND TESTS

Requested by Dr.:
Test for:
Prep:
Result:
Follow-up:

Requested by Dr.:
Test for:
Prep:
Result:
Follow-up:

Requested by Dr.:
Test for:
Prep:
Result:
Follow-up:

Requested by Dr.:
Test for:
Prep:
Result:
Follow-up:

TO-DO

Healing doesn't mean the damage never existed.
It means the damage no longer controls our lives.

— UNK

SUN/DOM	MON/LUN	TUES/MAR	WEDS/MIE	THURS/JUE	FRI/VIE	SAT/SA	

Notes

MONTH IN REVIEW

Current Meds

- ◇
- ◇
- ◇
- ◇
- ◇

New Meds

- ◇
- ◇
- ◇
- ◇
- ◇

Supplements

- ◇
- ◇
- ◇
- ◇
- ◇
- ◇

Reactions

- ◇
- ◇
- ◇
- ◇

Reactions

- ◇
- ◇
- ◇
- ◇

Reactions

- ◇
- ◇
- ◇
- ◇
- ◇
- ◇

NOTES

WOMEN'S HEALTH

Symptoms/Cycle

- ◇
- ◇
- ◇
- ◇

MEN'S HEALTH

Symptoms

- ◇
- ◇
- ◇
- ◇

QUESTIONS FOR YOUR CAREGIVER

Date/type of appointment:

_____

ANSWERS

Date/type of appointment:

_____

ANSWERS

Date/type of appointment:

_____

ANSWERS

NOTES

BLOOD WORK AND TESTS

Requested by Dr.:
Test for:
Prep:
Result:
Follow-up:

Requested by Dr.:
Test for:
Prep:
Result:
Follow-up:

Requested by Dr.:
Test for:
Prep:
Result:
Follow-up:

Requested by Dr.:
Test for:
Prep:
Result:
Follow-up:

TO-DO

Face the sunshine, and the shadows will fall behind. – UNK

SUN/DOM	MON/LUN	TUES/MAR	WEDS/MIE	THURS/JUE	FRI/VIE	SAT/SA

Notes

MONTH IN REVIEW

Current Meds
- ▷
- ▷
- ▷
- ▷

New Meds
- ▷
- ▷
- ▷
- ▷

Supplements
- ▷
- ▷
- ▷
- ▷
- ▷
- ▷

Reactions
- ▷
- ▷
- ▷
- ▷

Reactions
- ▷
- ▷
- ▷
- ▷

Reactions
- ▷
- ▷
- ▷
- ▷
- ▷

NOTES

WOMEN'S HEALTH

Symptoms/Cycle
- ▷
- ▷
- ▷
- ▷

MEN'S HEALTH

Symptoms
- ▷
- ▷
- ▷
- ▷

QUESTIONS FOR YOUR CAREGIVER

Date/type of appointment:

_____

ANSWERS

Date/type of appointment:

_____

ANSWERS

Date/type of appointment:

_____

ANSWERS

NOTES

BLOOD WORK AND TESTS

Requested by Dr.:
Test for:
Prep:
Result:
Follow-up:

Requested by Dr.:
Test for:
Prep:
Result:
Follow-up:

Requested by Dr.:
Test for:
Prep:
Result:
Follow-up:

Requested by Dr.:
Test for:
Prep:
Result:
Follow-up:

TO-DO

*You will always have bad times,
but they will always wake you up to the
stuff you weren't paying attention to.*
— ROBIN WILLIAMS

SUN/DOM	MON/LUN	TUES/MAR	WEDS/MIE	THURS/JUE	FRI/VIE	SAT/SA

Notes

MONTH IN REVIEW

Current Meds
▷ ▷ ▷ ▷
▷ ▷ ▷ ▷

New Meds
▷ ▷ ▷ ▷
▷ ▷ ▷ ▷

Supplements
▷ ▷ ▷ ▷ ▷ ▷
▷ ▷

Reactions
▷ ▷ ▷ ▷
▷ ▷ ▷ ▷

Reactions
▷ ▷ ▷ ▷
▷ ▷ ▷ ▷

Reactions
▷ ▷ ▷ ▷ ▷
▷ ▷ ▷

NOTES

WOMEN'S HEALTH

Symptoms/Cycle
▷ ▷ ▷ ▷

MEN'S HEALTH

Symptoms
▷ ▷ ▷ ▷

QUESTIONS FOR YOUR CAREGIVER

Date/type of appointment:

_____

ANSWERS

Date/type of appointment:

_____

ANSWERS

Date/type of appointment:

_____

ANSWERS

NOTES

BLOOD WORK AND TESTS

Requested by Dr.:
Test for:
Prep:
Result:
Follow-up:

Requested by Dr.:
Test for:
Prep:
Result:
Follow-up:

Requested by Dr.:
Test for:
Prep:
Result:
Follow-up:

Requested by Dr.:
Test for:
Prep:
Result:
Follow-up:

TO-DO

The art of ritual and self care is
available to you anytime, anywhere.
— JEANNIE JARNOT

SUN/DOM	MON/LUN	TUES/MAR	WEDS/MIE	THURS/JUE	FRI/VIE	SAT/SA	

Notes

MONTH IN REVIEW

Current Meds
- ▷
- ▷
- ▷
- ▷
- ▷

New Meds
- ▷
- ▷
- ▷
- ▷

Supplements
- ▷
- ▷
- ▷
- ▷
- ▷
- ▷
- ▷

Reactions
- ▷
- ▷
- ▷
- ▷
- ▷

Reactions
- ▷
- ▷
- ▷
- ▷
- ▷

Reactions
- ▷
- ▷
- ▷
- ▷
- ▷
- ▷

NOTES

WOMEN'S HEALTH

Symptoms/Cycle
- ▷
- ▷
- ▷
- ▷

MEN'S HEALTH

Symptoms
- ▷
- ▷
- ▷
- ▷

QUESTIONS FOR YOUR CAREGIVER

Date/type of appointment:

_____

ANSWERS

Date/type of appointment:

_____

ANSWERS

Date/type of appointment:

_____

ANSWERS

NOTES

BLOOD WORK AND TESTS

Requested by Dr.:
Test for:
Prep:
Result:
Follow-up:

Requested by Dr.:
Test for:
Prep:
Result:
Follow-up:

Requested by Dr.:
Test for:
Prep:
Result:
Follow-up:

Requested by Dr.:
Test for:
Prep:
Result:
Follow-up:

TO-DO

If I cannot do great things,
I can do small things in a great way.
— MARTIN LUTHER KING JR.

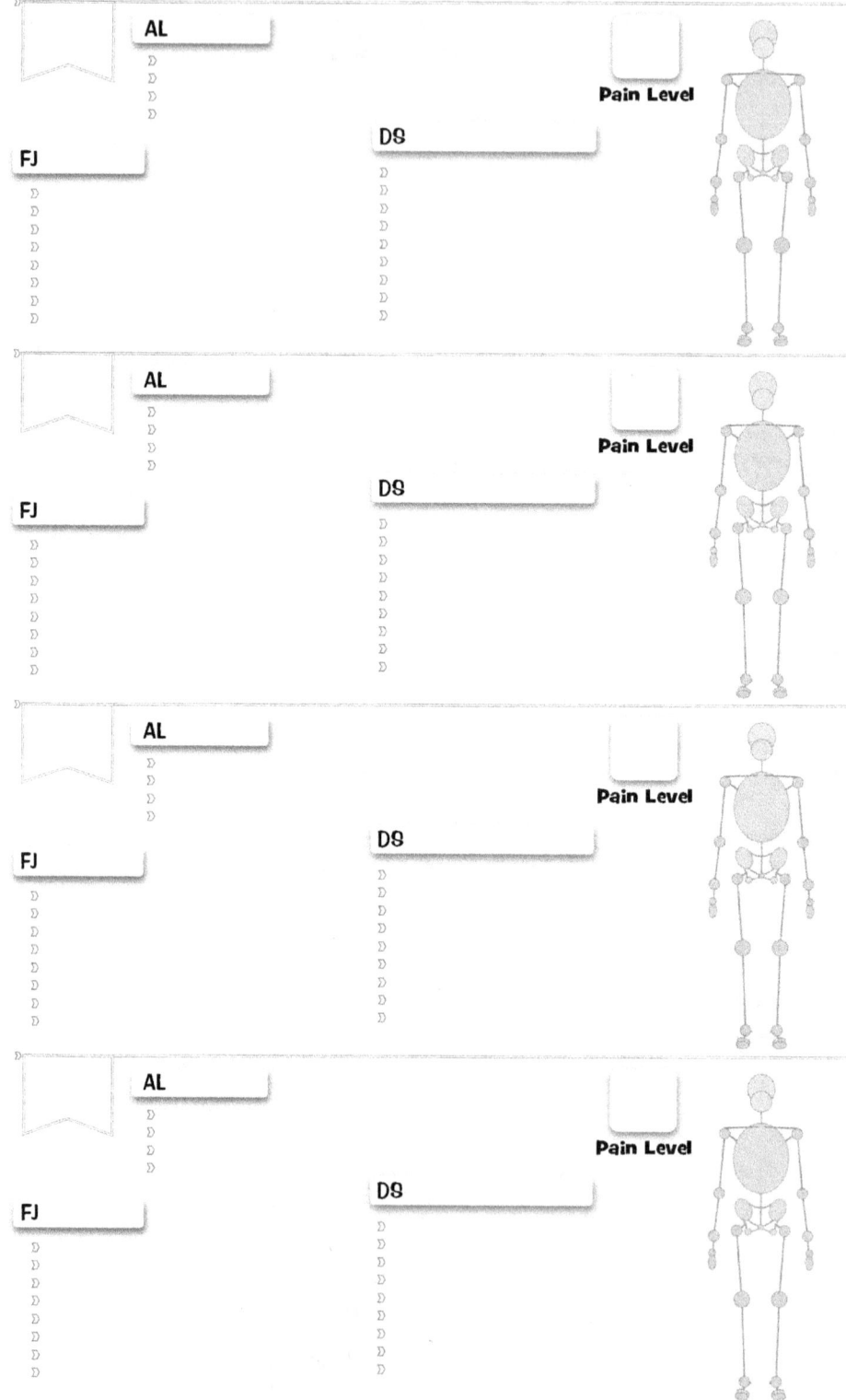

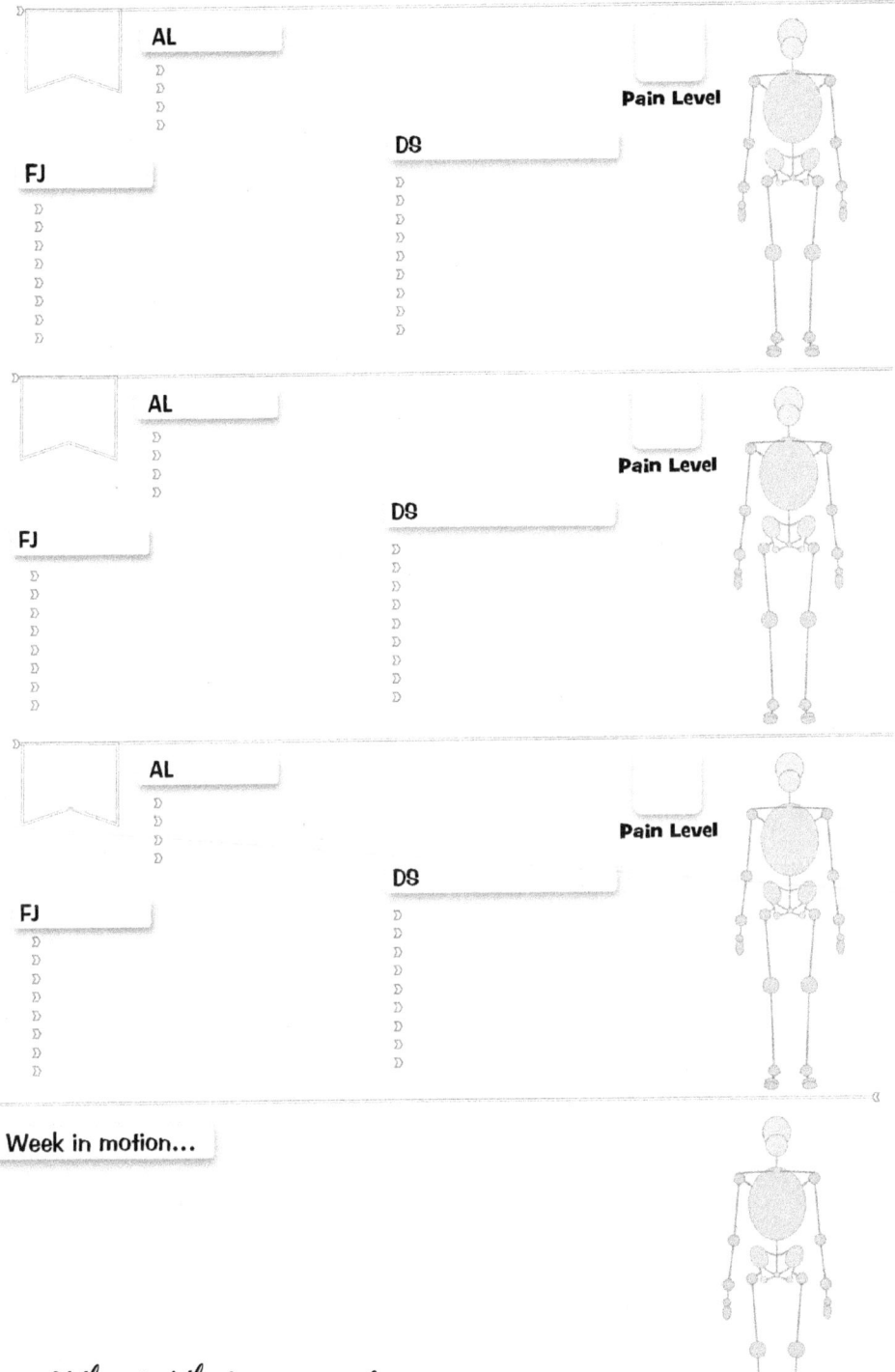

AL

Pain Level

DS

FJ

AL

Pain Level

DS

FJ

AL

Pain Level

DS

FJ

Week in motion...

At the end of the day, we can endure
much more than we think we can.
— FRIDA KAHLO

R   **L**

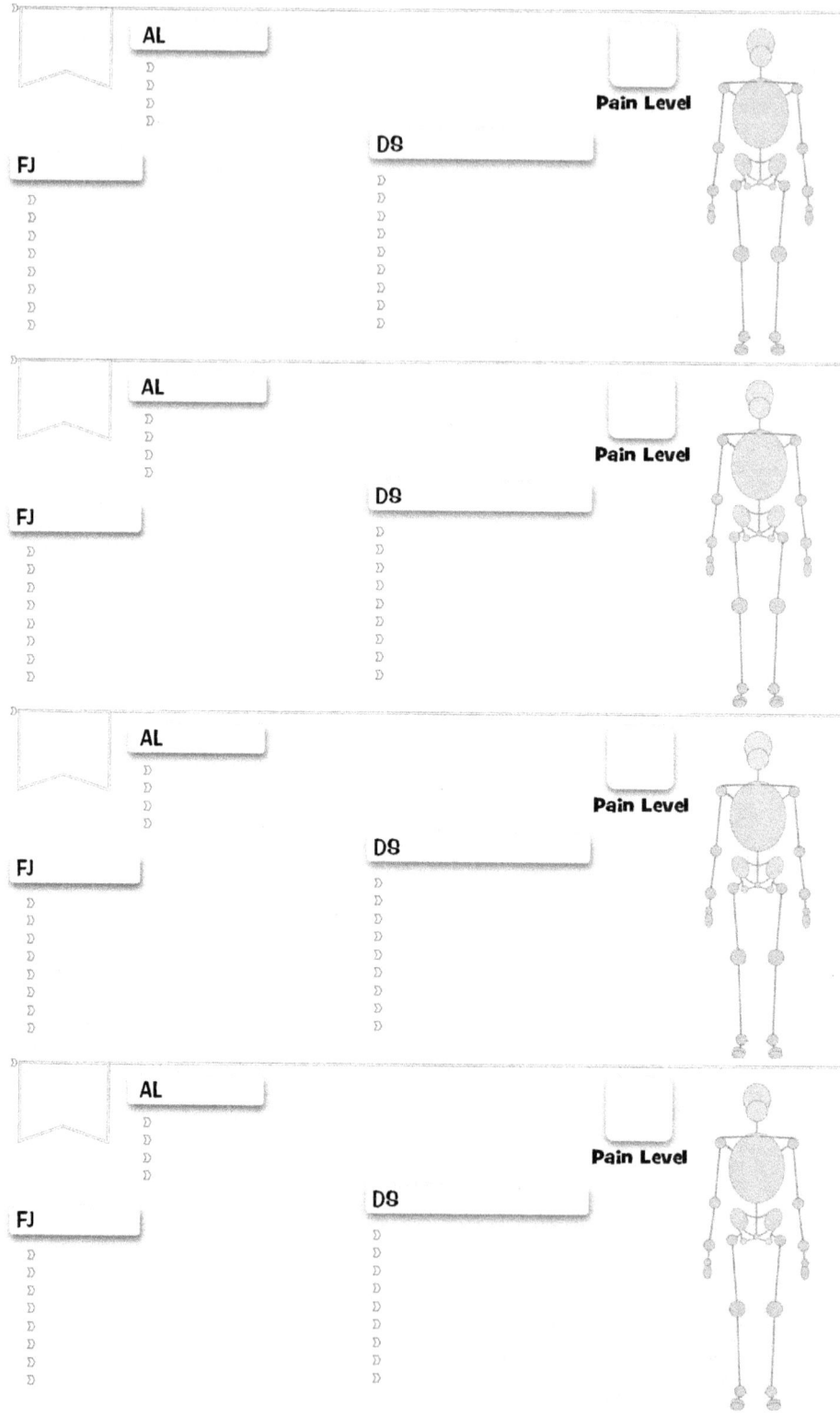

AL

FJ

DS

Pain Level

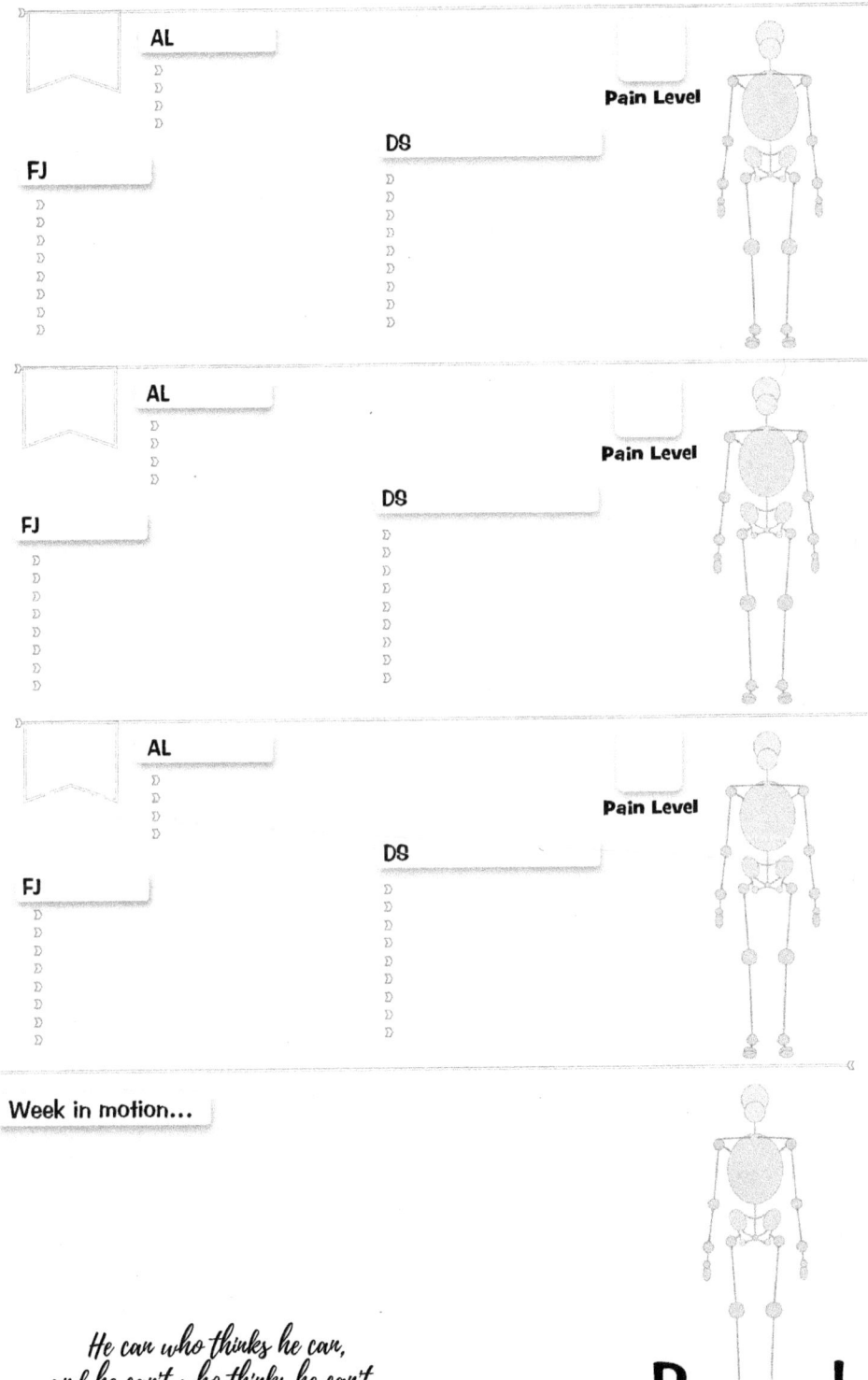

AL

Pain Level

FJ

DS

AL

Pain Level

FJ

DS

AL

Pain Level

FJ

DS

Week in motion...

He can who thinks he can,
and he can't who thinks he can't .
— PABLO PICASSO

R   **L**

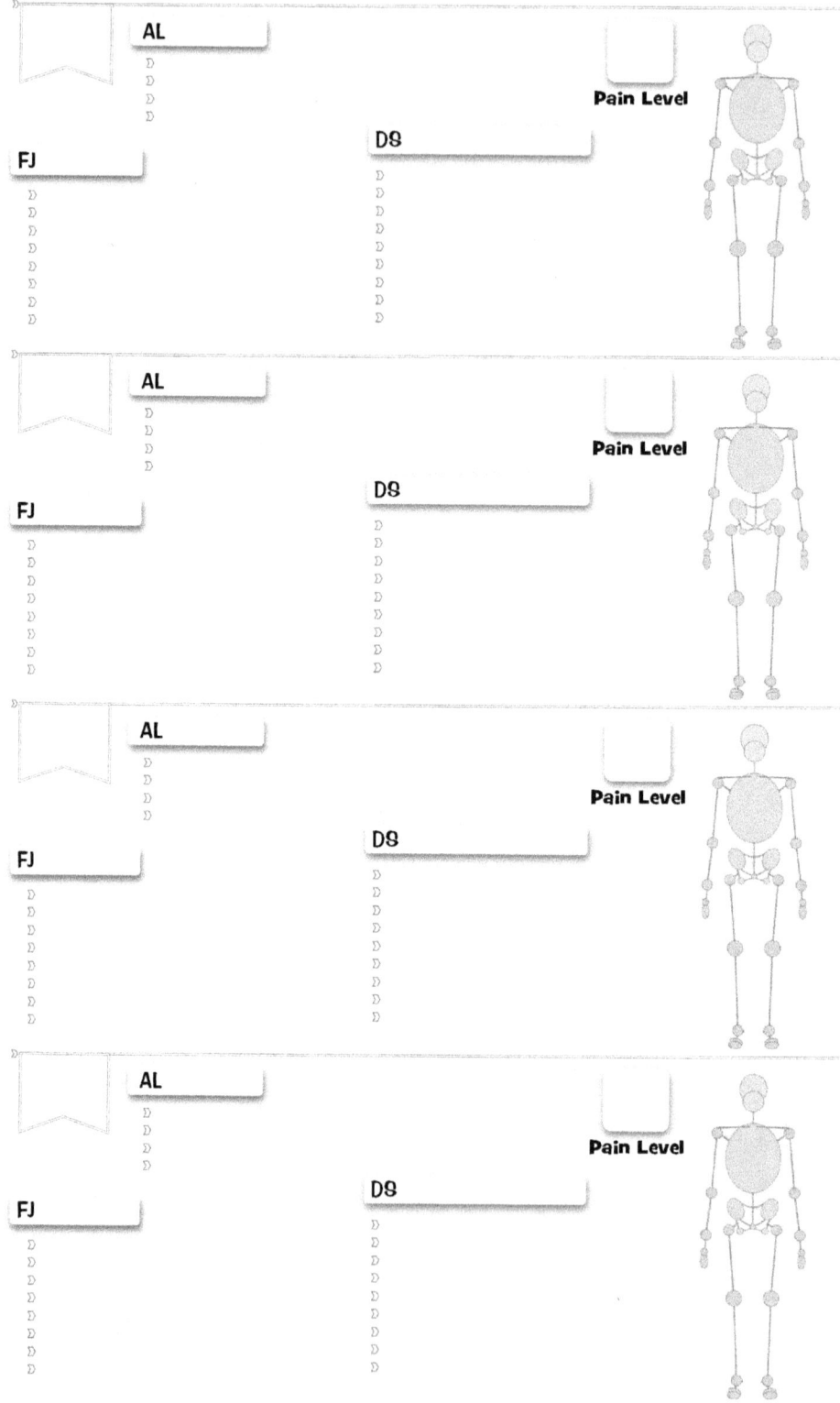

AL

FJ

DS

Pain Level

AL

FJ

DS

Pain Level

AL

FJ

DS

Pain Level

AL

FJ

DS

Pain Level

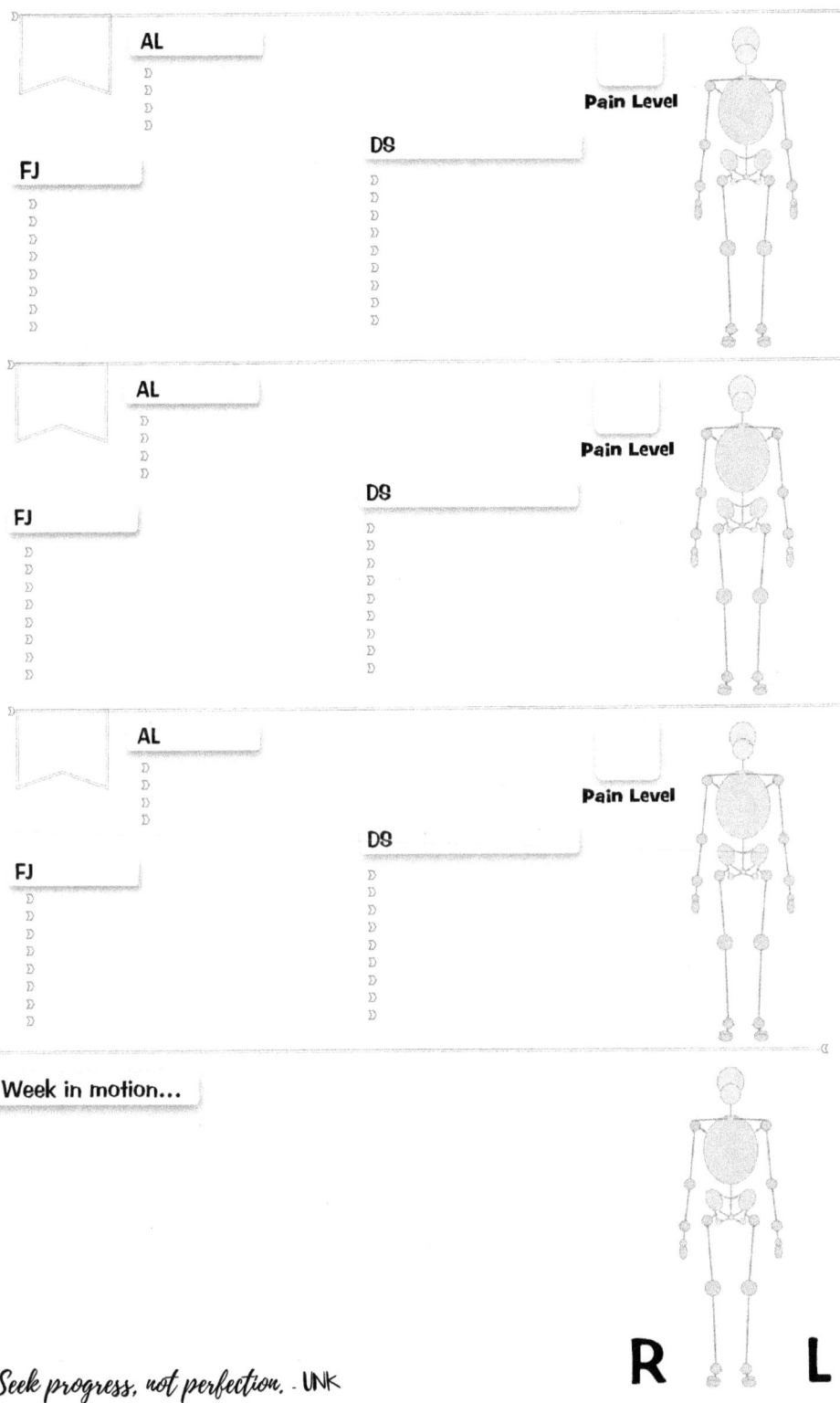

AL

Pain Level

DS

FJ

AL

Pain Level

DS

FJ

AL

DS

Pain Level

FJ

Week in motion...

Seek progress, not perfection. - UNK

R **L**

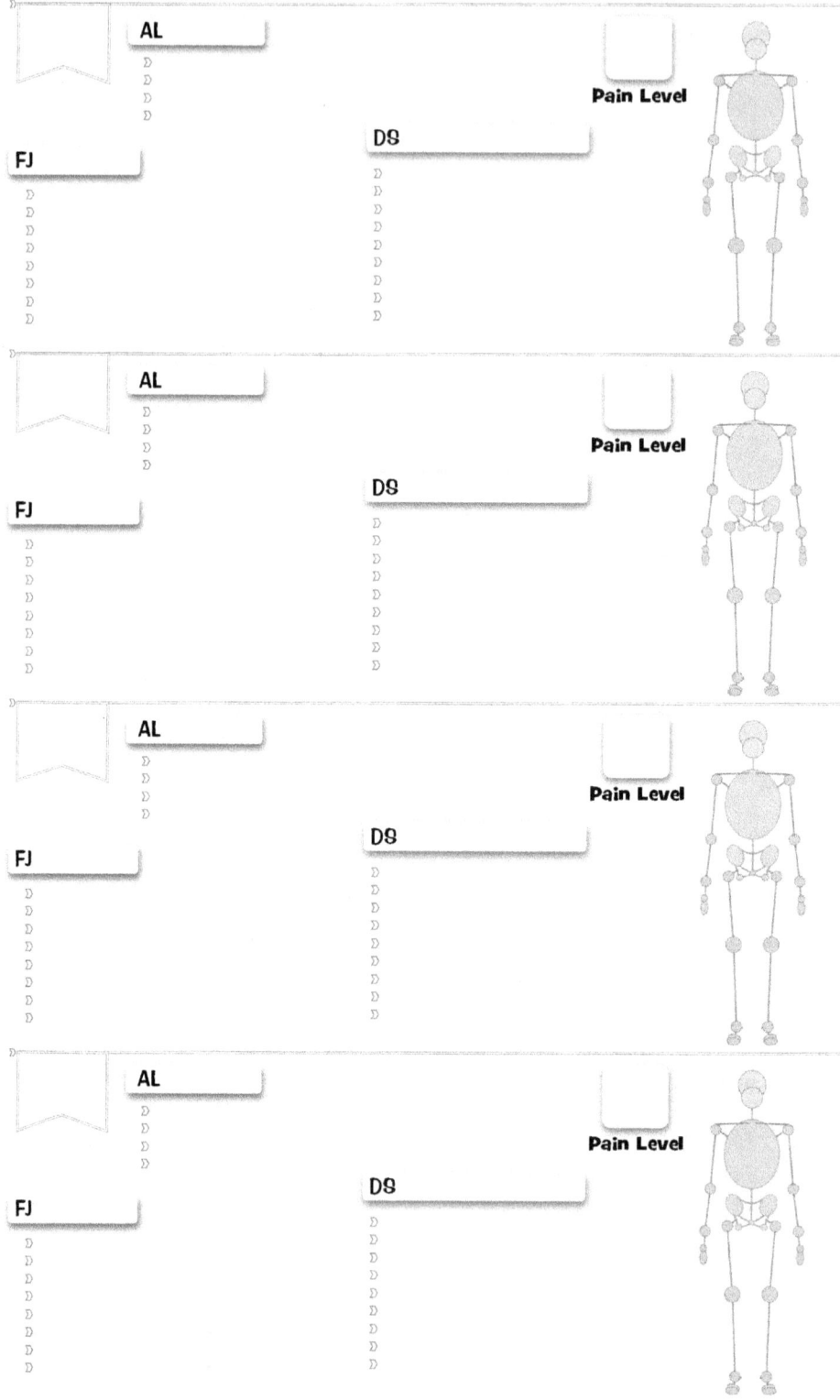

AL

FJ

DS

Pain Level

AL

FJ

DS

Pain Level

AL

FJ

DS

Pain Level

AL

FJ

DS

Pain Level

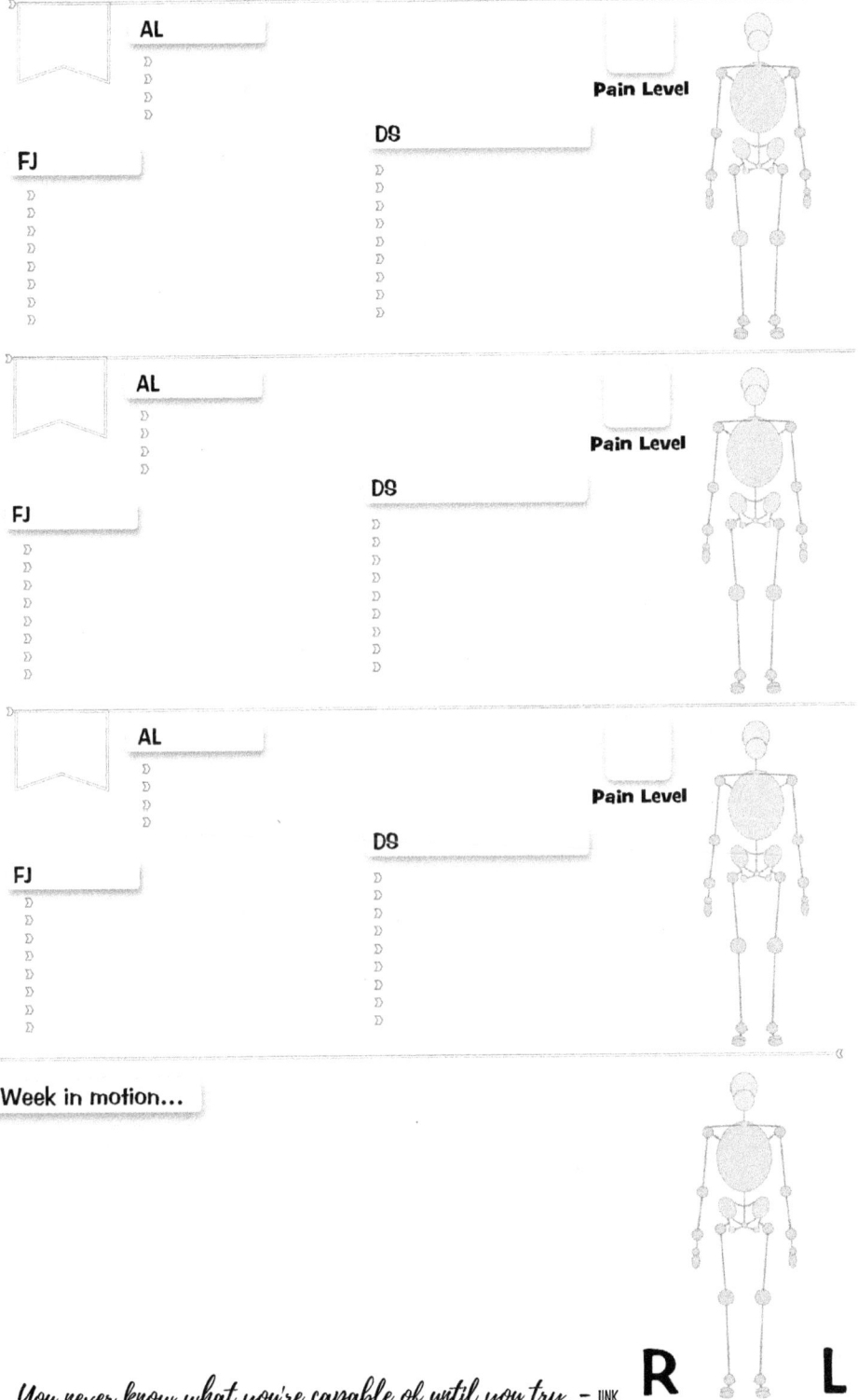

AL
>
>
>

FJ
>
>
>
>
>
>

DS
>
>
>
>
>
>

Pain Level

AL
>
>
>

FJ
>
>
>
>
>
>

DS
>
>
>
>
>
>

Pain Level

AL
>
>
>

FJ
>
>
>
>
>
>

DS
>
>
>
>
>
>

Pain Level

Week in motion...

You never know what you're capable of until you try. – UNK

R　　**L**

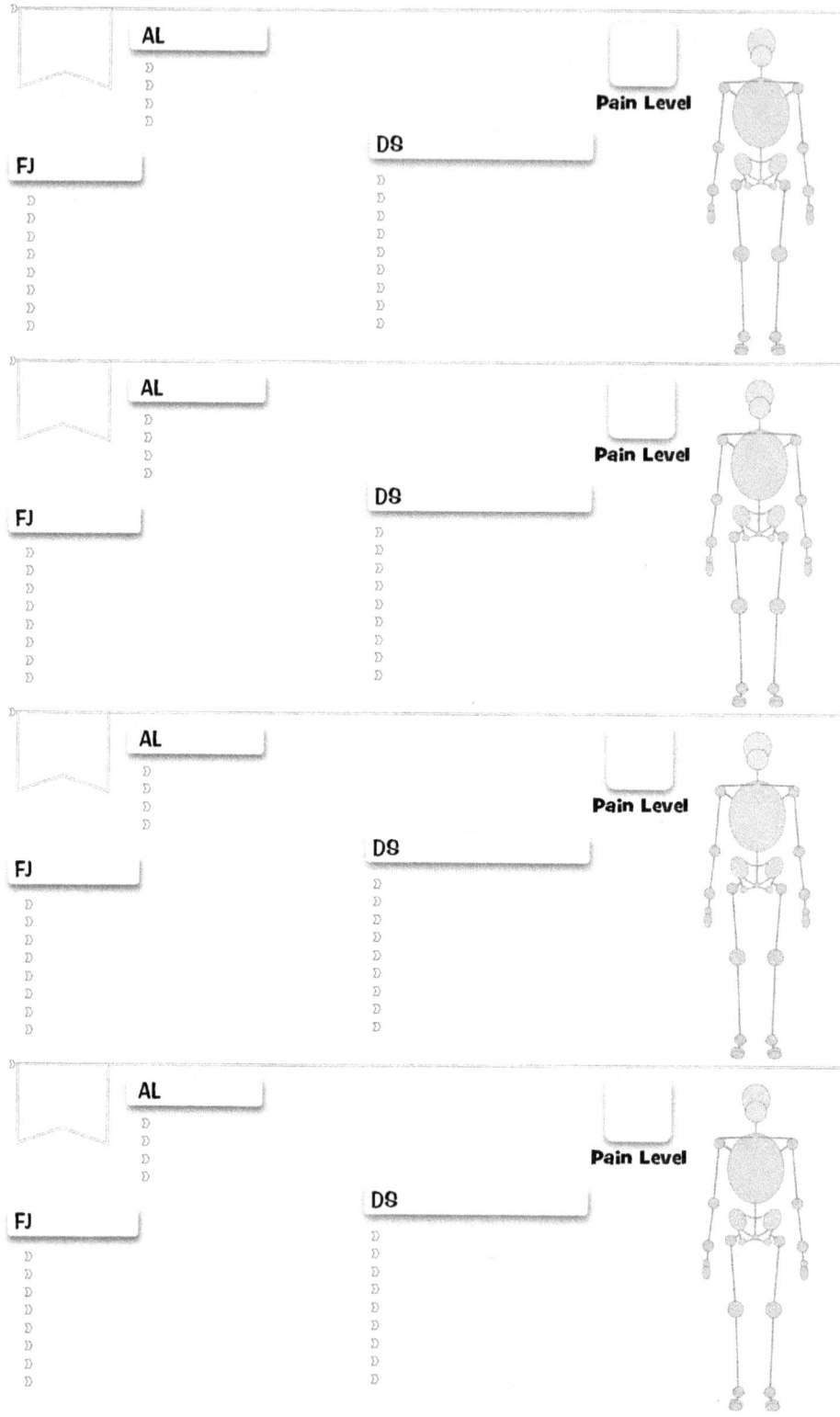

AL

FJ

DS

Pain Level

AL

FJ

DS

Pain Level

AL

FJ

DS

Pain Level

AL

FJ

DS

Pain Level

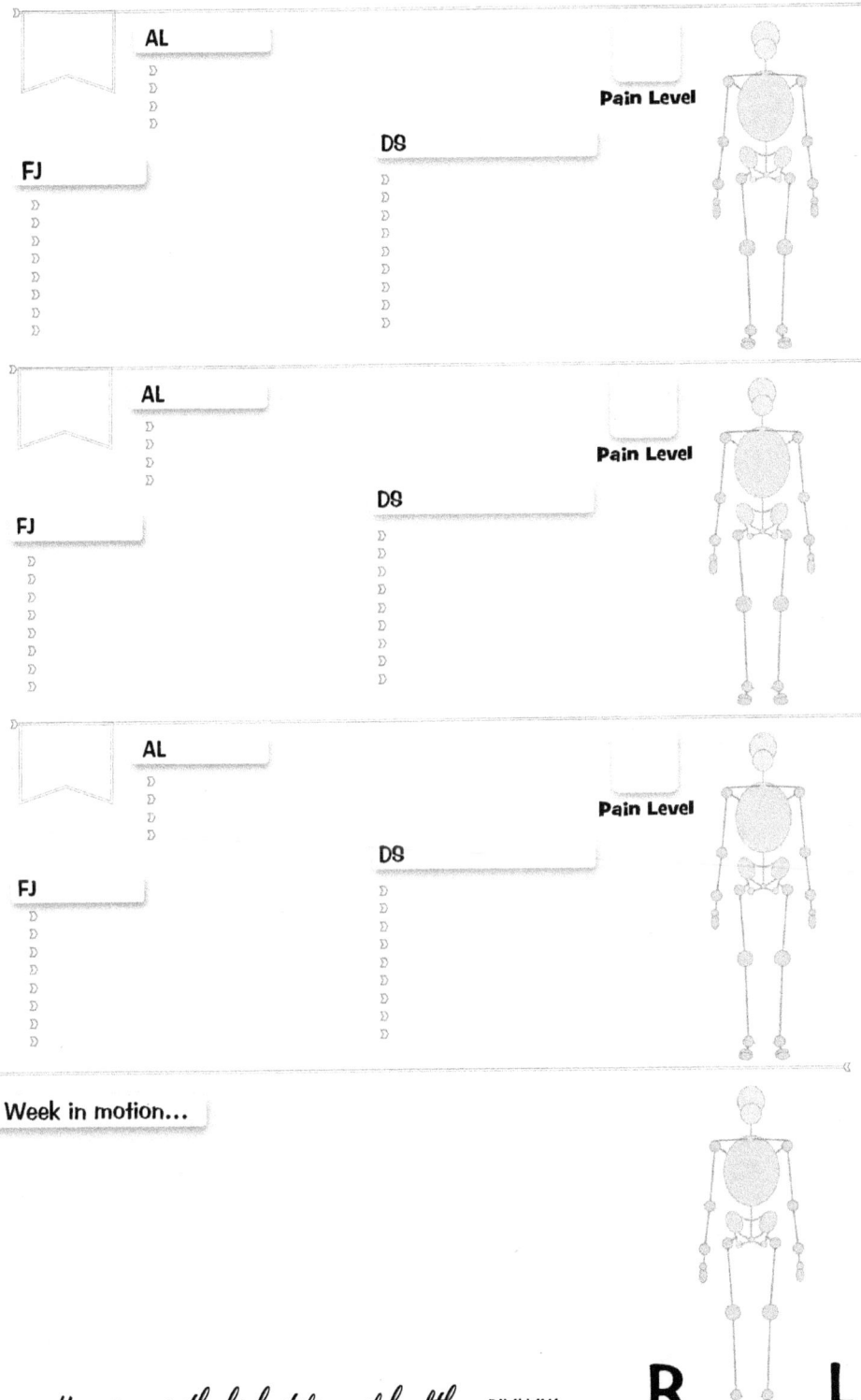

AL

Pain Level

DS

FJ

AL

Pain Level

DS

FJ

AL

Pain Level

DS

FJ

Week in motion...

Happiness is the highest form of health. – DALAI LAMA

R   **L**

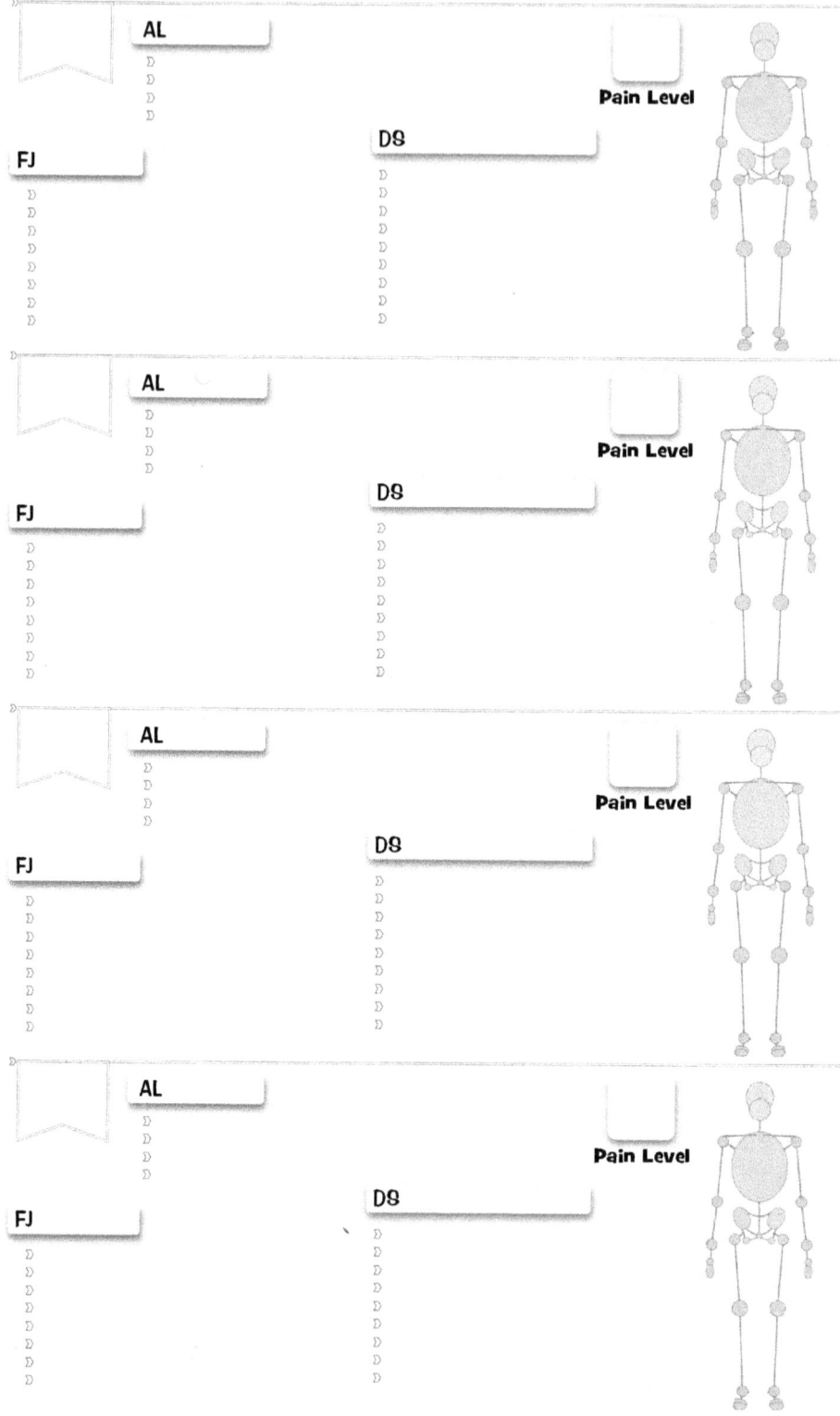

AL

FJ

DS

Pain Level

AL

FJ

DS

Pain Level

AL

FJ

DS

Pain Level

AL

FJ

DS

Pain Level

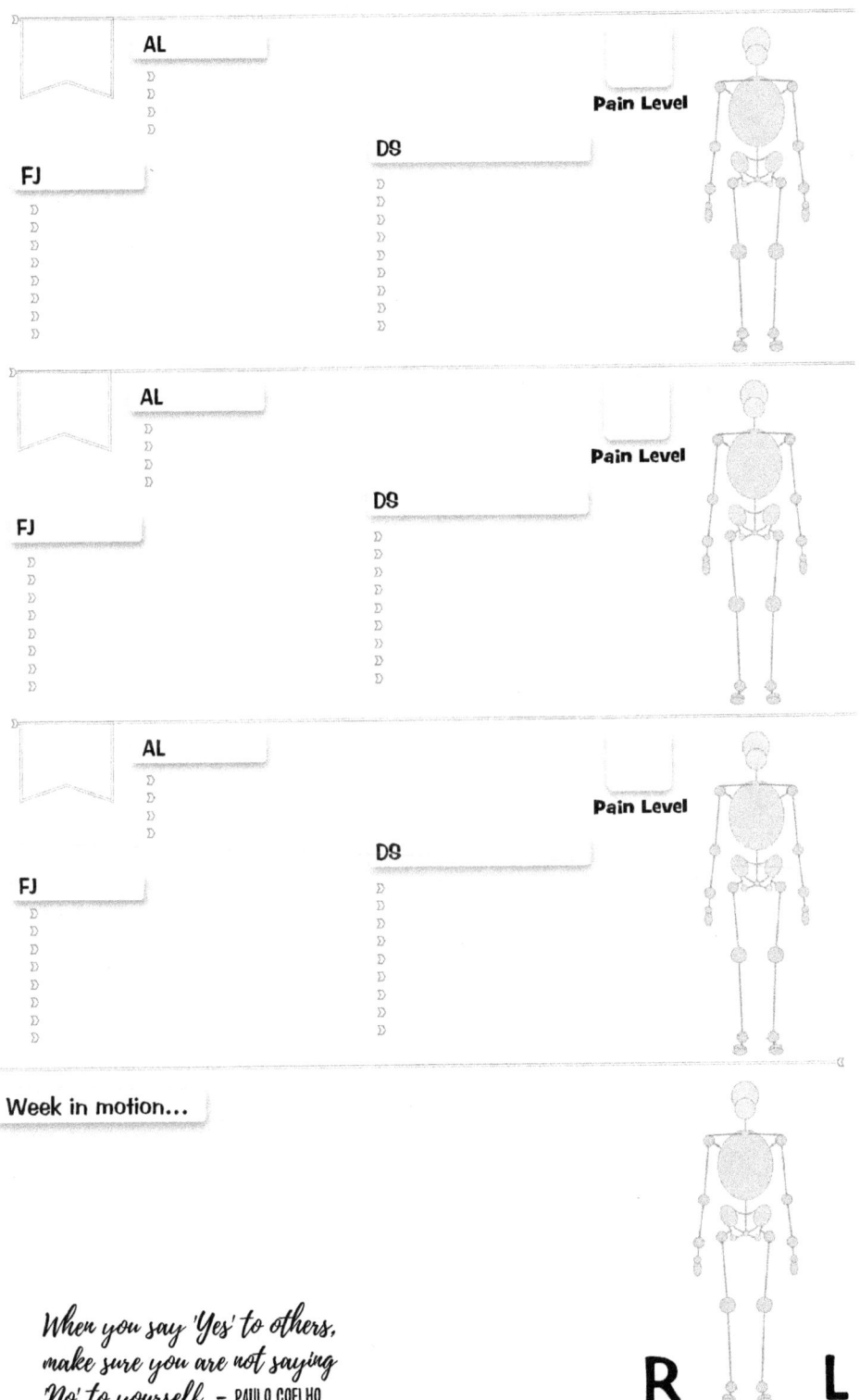

AL

Pain Level

FJ

DS

AL

Pain Level

FJ

DS

AL

Pain Level

FJ

DS

Week in motion...

When you say 'Yes' to others, make sure you are not saying 'No' to yourself. – PAULO COELHO

R   **L**

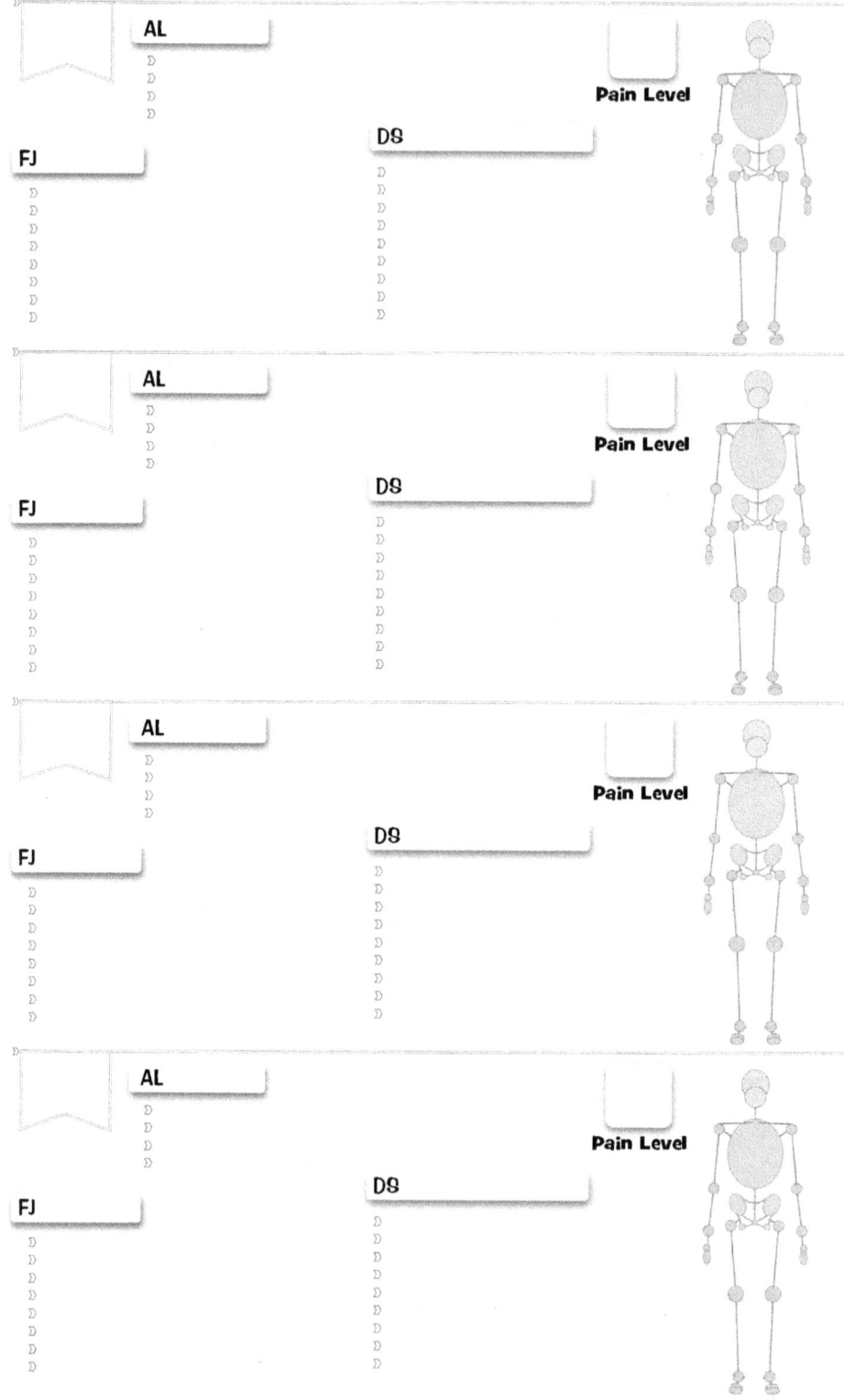

AL

FJ

DS

Pain Level

AL

FJ

DS

Pain Level

AL

FJ

DS

Pain Level

AL

FJ

DS

Pain Level

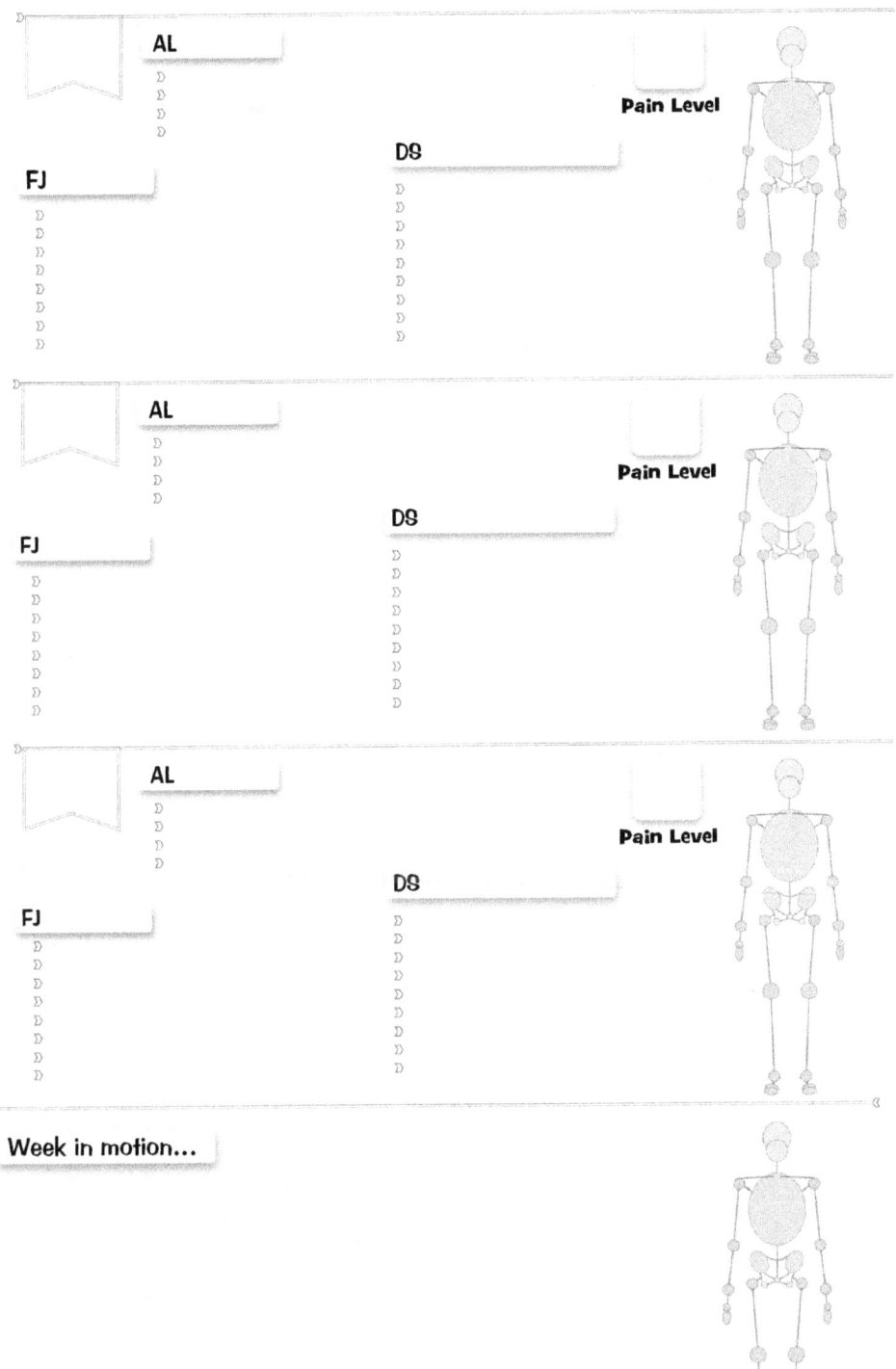

AL

Pain Level

FJ

DS

AL

Pain Level

FJ

DS

AL

Pain Level

FJ

DS

Week in motion...

*Make sure your worst enemy doesn't
live between your own two ears.*
— LAIRD HAMILTON

R   **L**

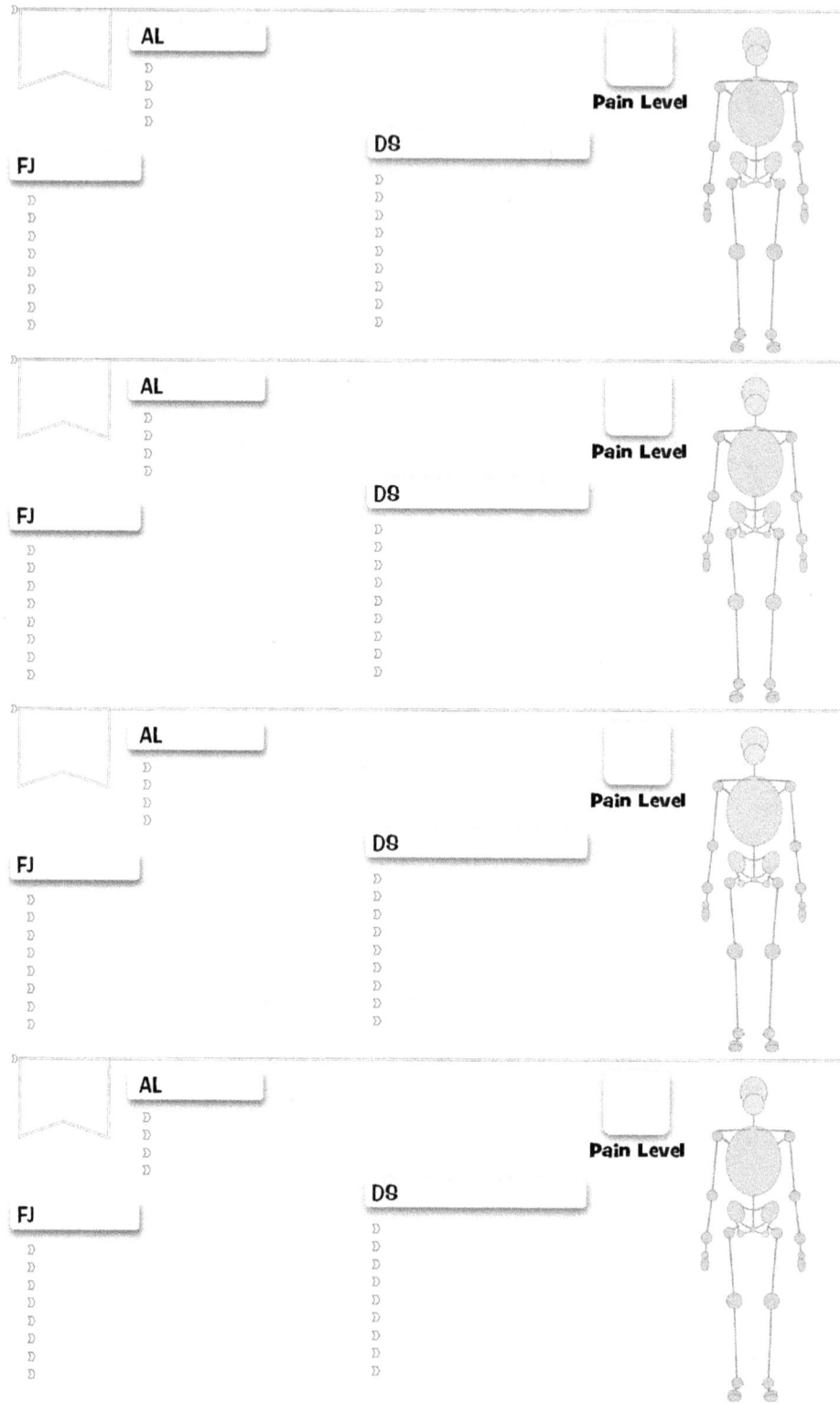

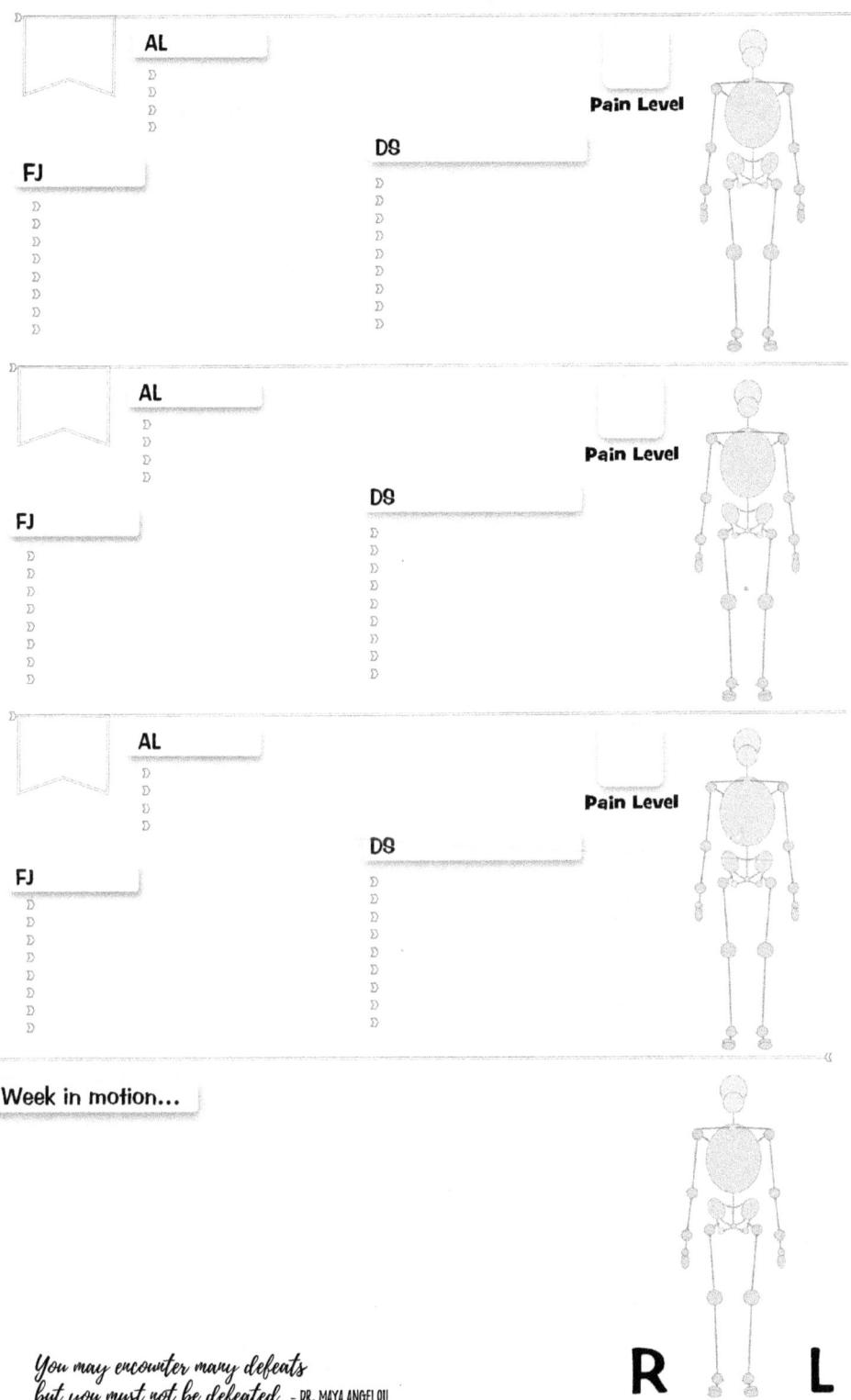

AL
- ꒿
- ꒿
- ꒿
- ꒿

FJ
- ꒿
- ꒿
- ꒿
- ꒿
- ꒿
- ꒿
- ꒿

DS
- ꒿
- ꒿
- ꒿
- ꒿
- ꒿
- ꒿
- ꒿

Pain Level

AL
- ꒿
- ꒿
- ꒿

FJ
- ꒿
- ꒿
- ꒿
- ꒿
- ꒿
- ꒿

DS
- ꒿
- ꒿
- ꒿
- ꒿
- ꒿
- ꒿
- ꒿

Pain Level

AL
- ꒿
- ꒿
- ꒿

FJ
- ꒿
- ꒿
- ꒿
- ꒿
- ꒿
- ꒿

DS
- ꒿
- ꒿
- ꒿
- ꒿
- ꒿
- ꒿

Pain Level

Week in motion...

You may encounter many defeats but you must not be defeated. – DR. MAYA ANGELOU

R   **L**

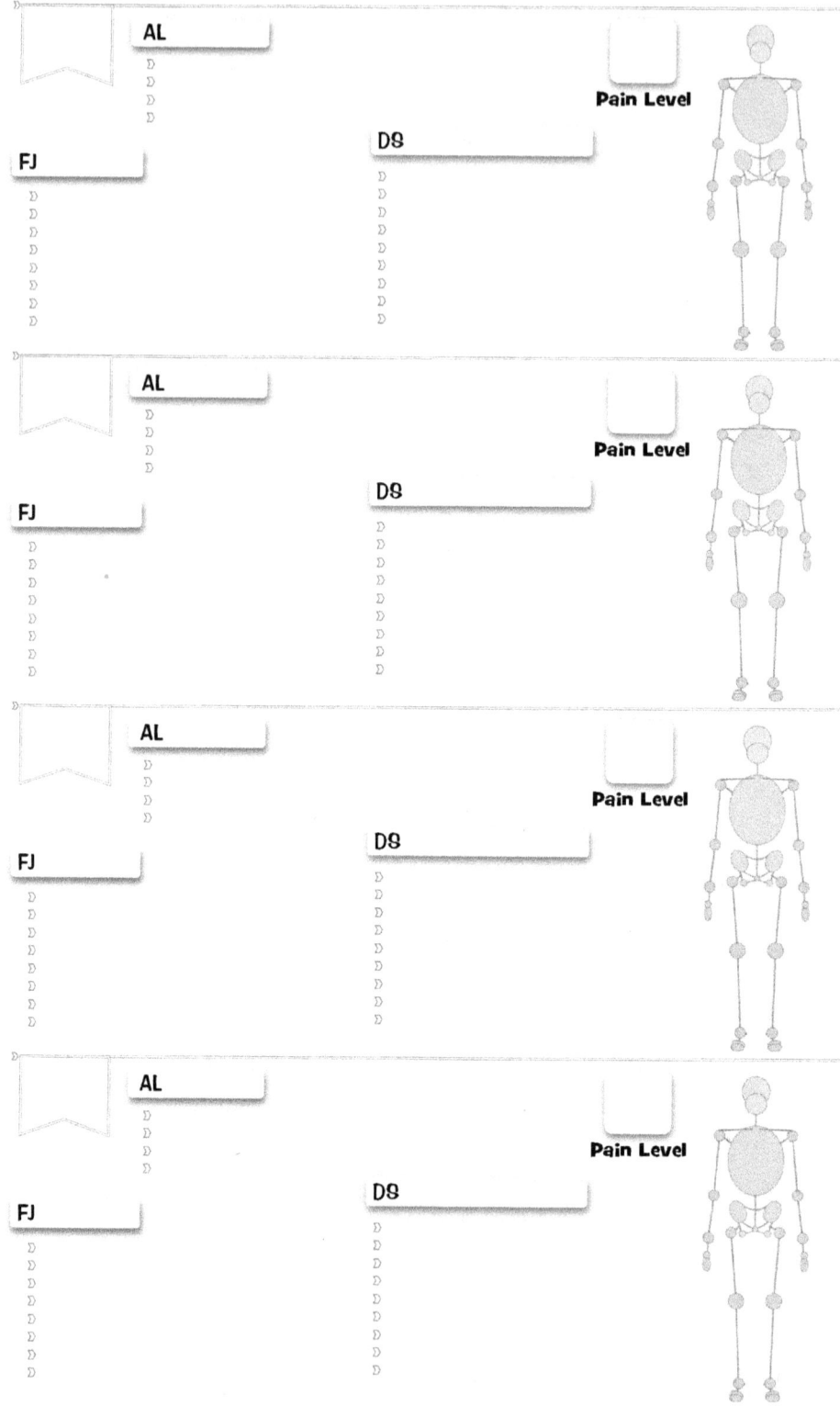

AL

FJ

DS

Pain Level

AL

FJ

DS

Pain Level

AL

FJ

DS

Pain Level

AL

FJ

DS

Pain Level

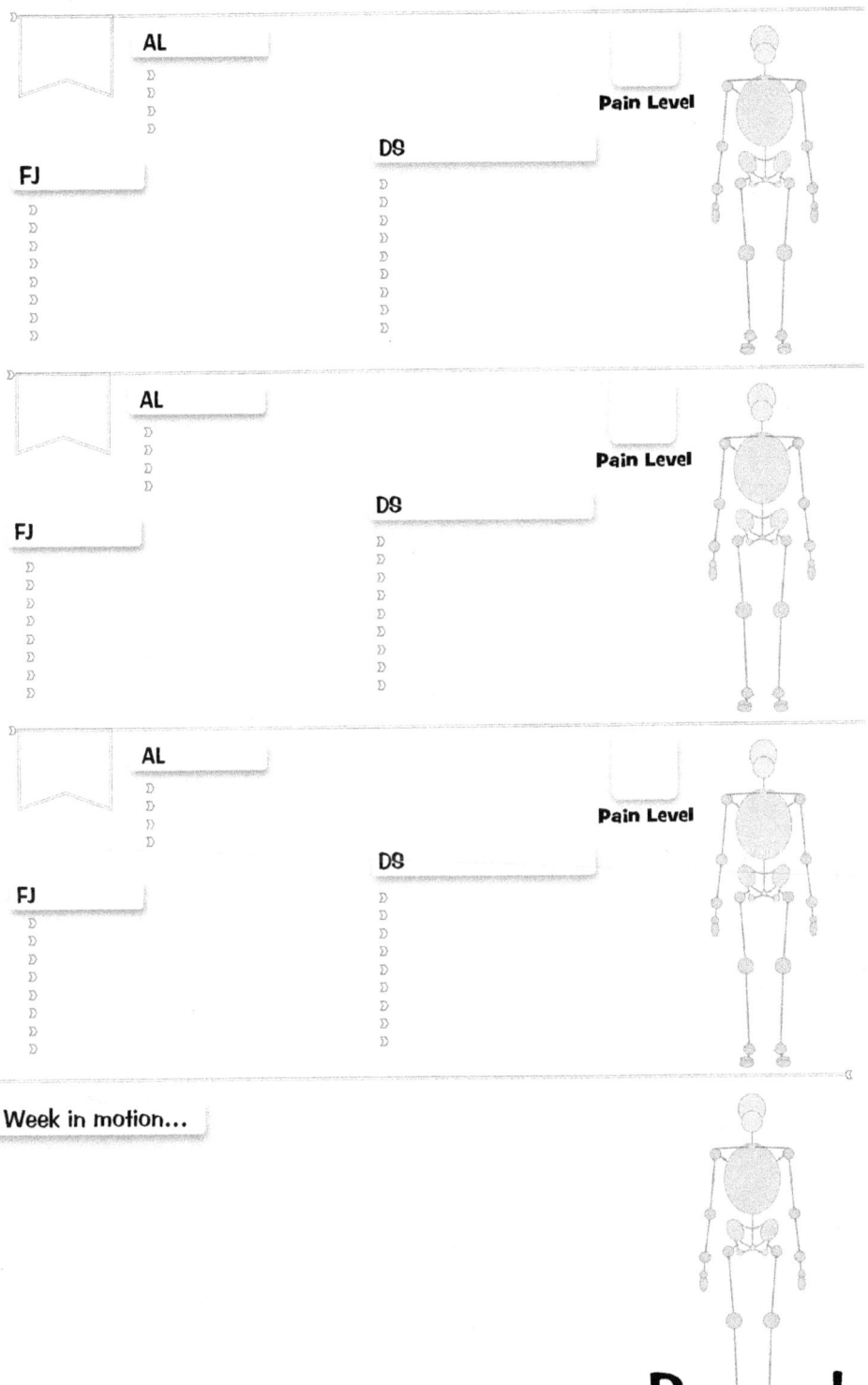

AL

Pain Level

FJ

DS

AL

Pain Level

FJ

DS

AL

Pain Level

FJ

DS

Week in motion...

R   L

Do you live to work, or work to live?

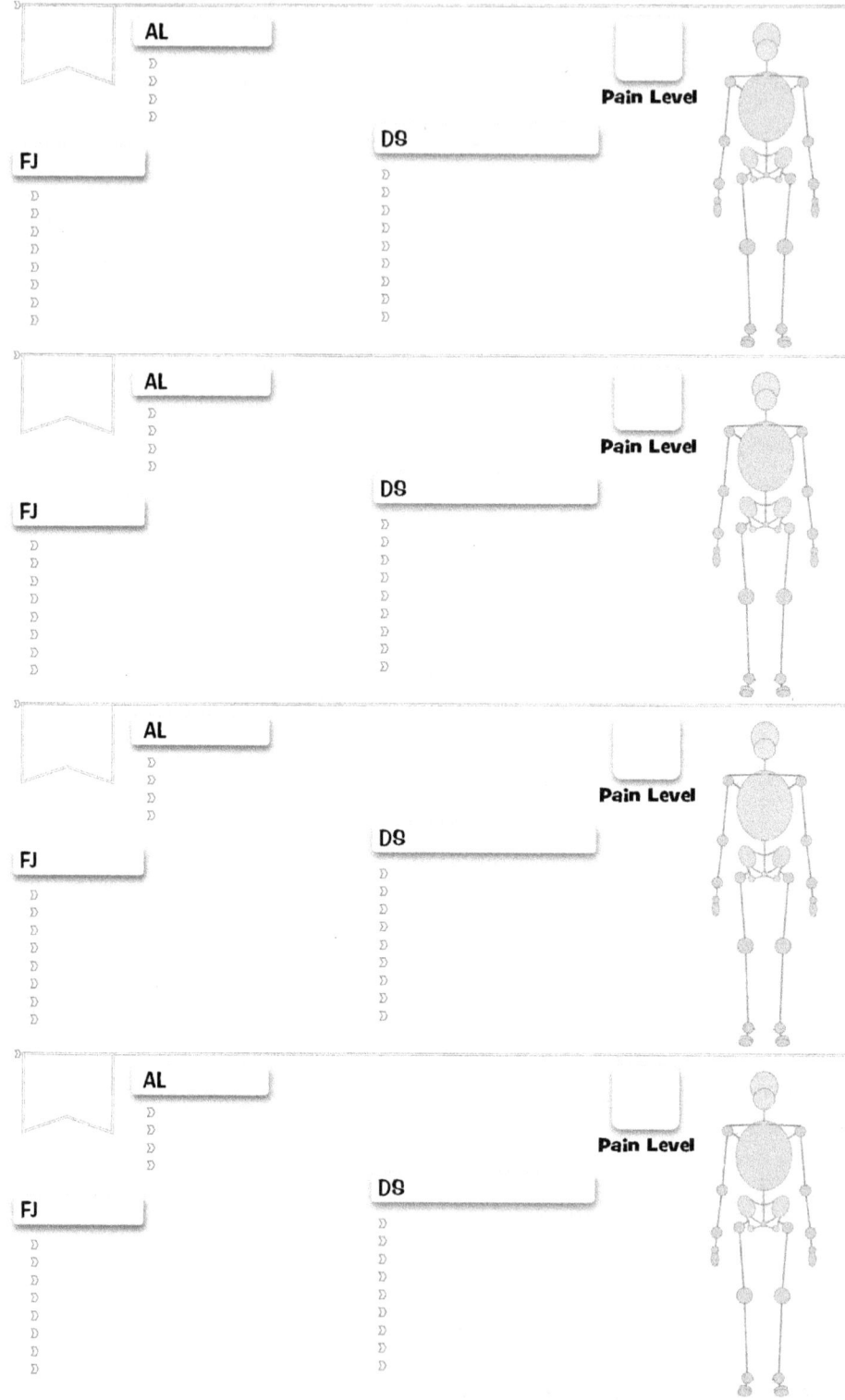

AL

FJ

DS

Pain Level

AL

FJ

DS

Pain Level

AL

FJ

DS

Pain Level

AL

FJ

DS

Pain Level

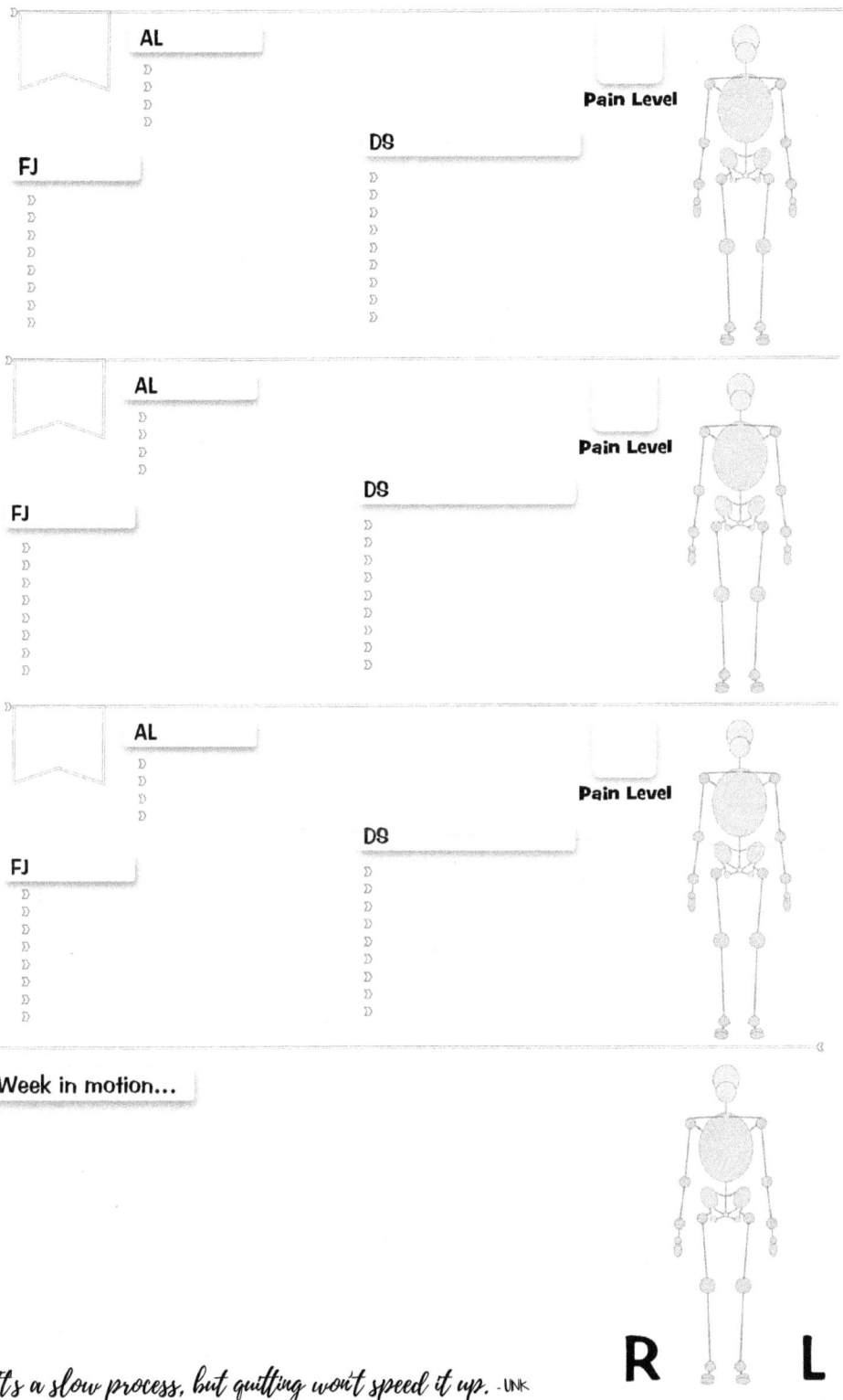

AL

FJ

DS

Pain Level

AL

Pain Level

DS

FJ

AL

Pain Level

DS

FJ

Week in motion...

R   **L**

It's a slow process, but quitting won't speed it up. -UNK

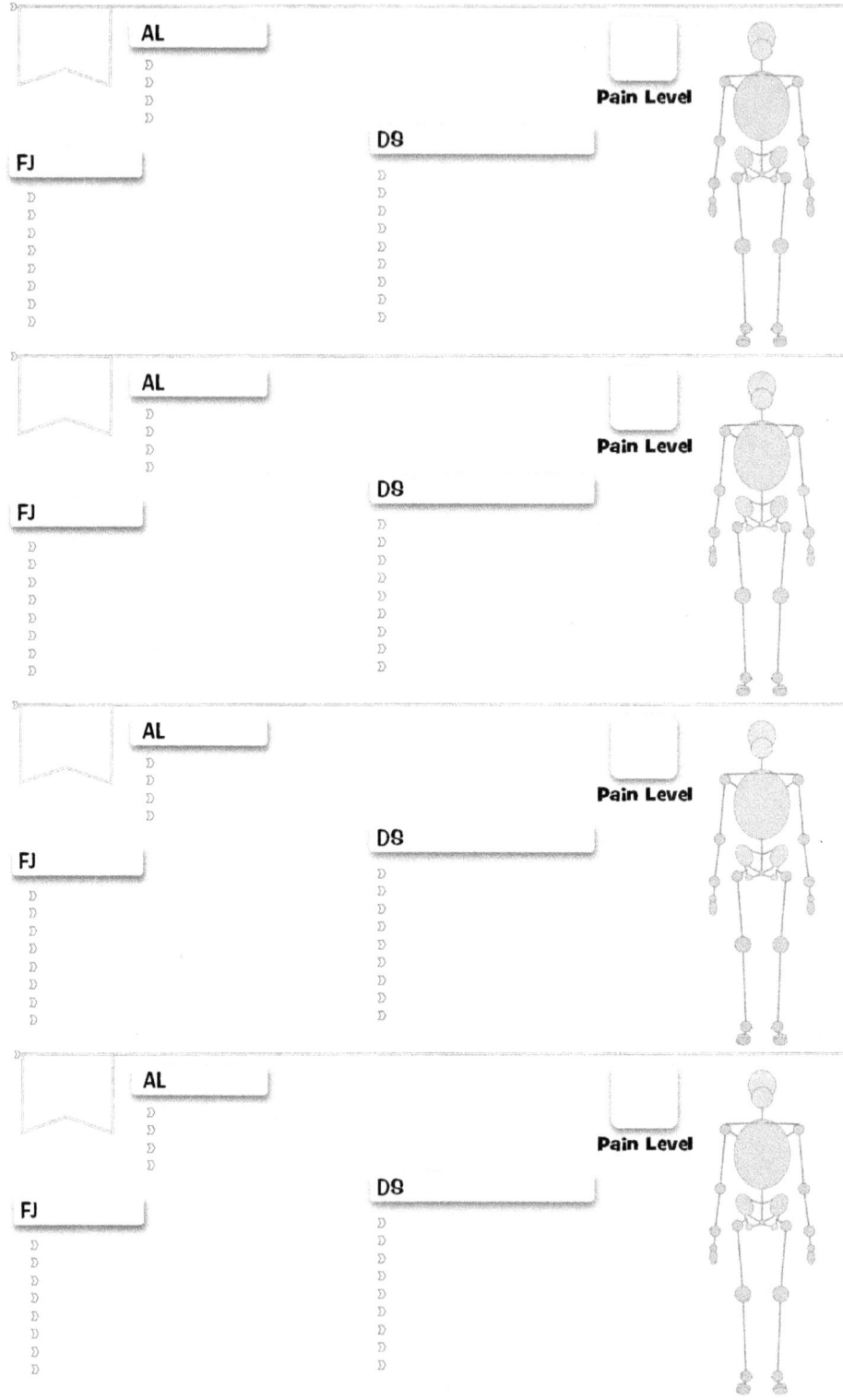

AL

FJ

Pain Level

DS

AL

FJ

Pain Level

DS

AL

FJ

Pain Level

DS

AL

FJ

Pain Level

DS

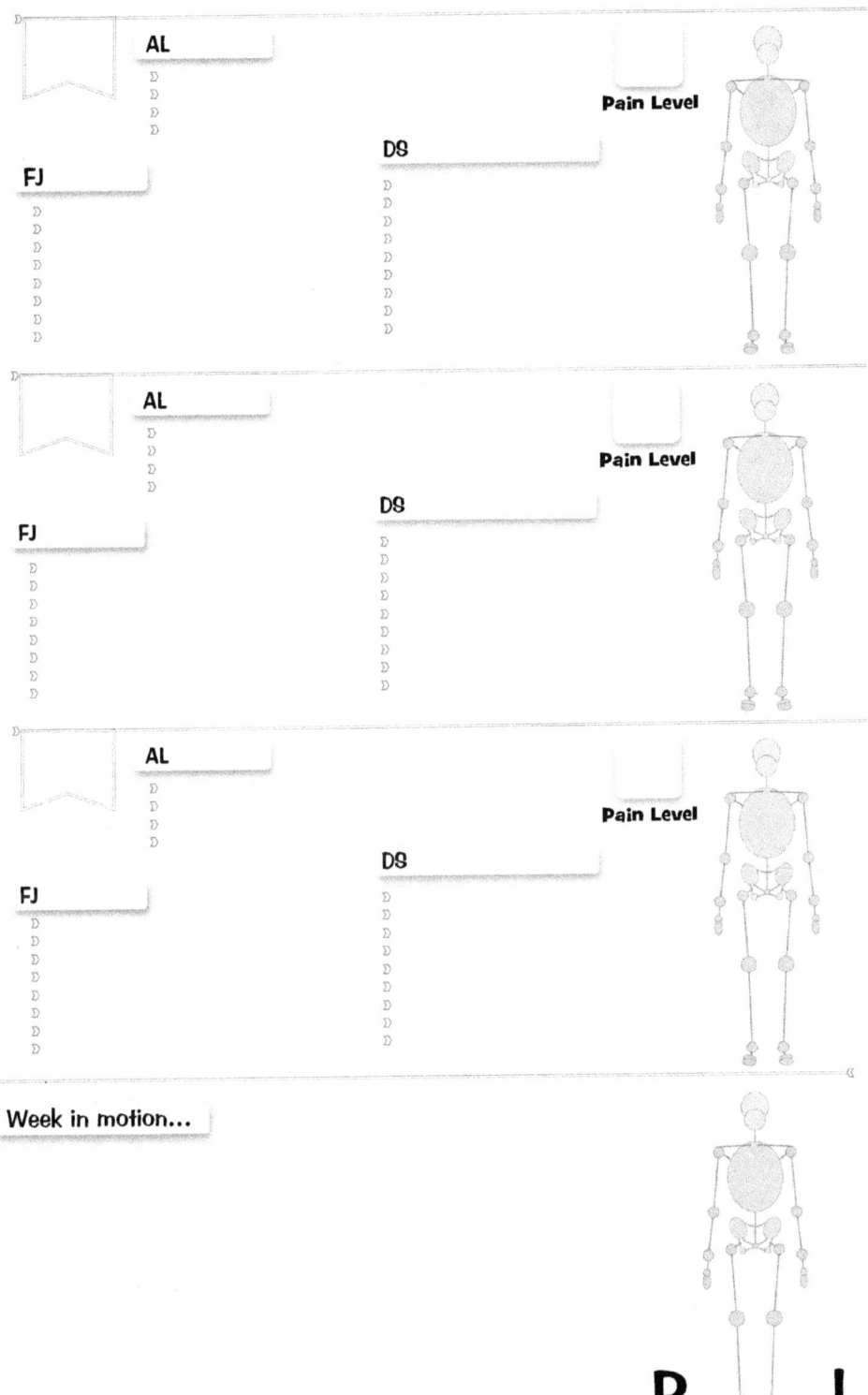

AL

FJ

DS

Pain Level

AL

FJ

DS

Pain Level

AL

FJ

DS

Pain Level

Week in motion...

R   L

It is NOT in your head.

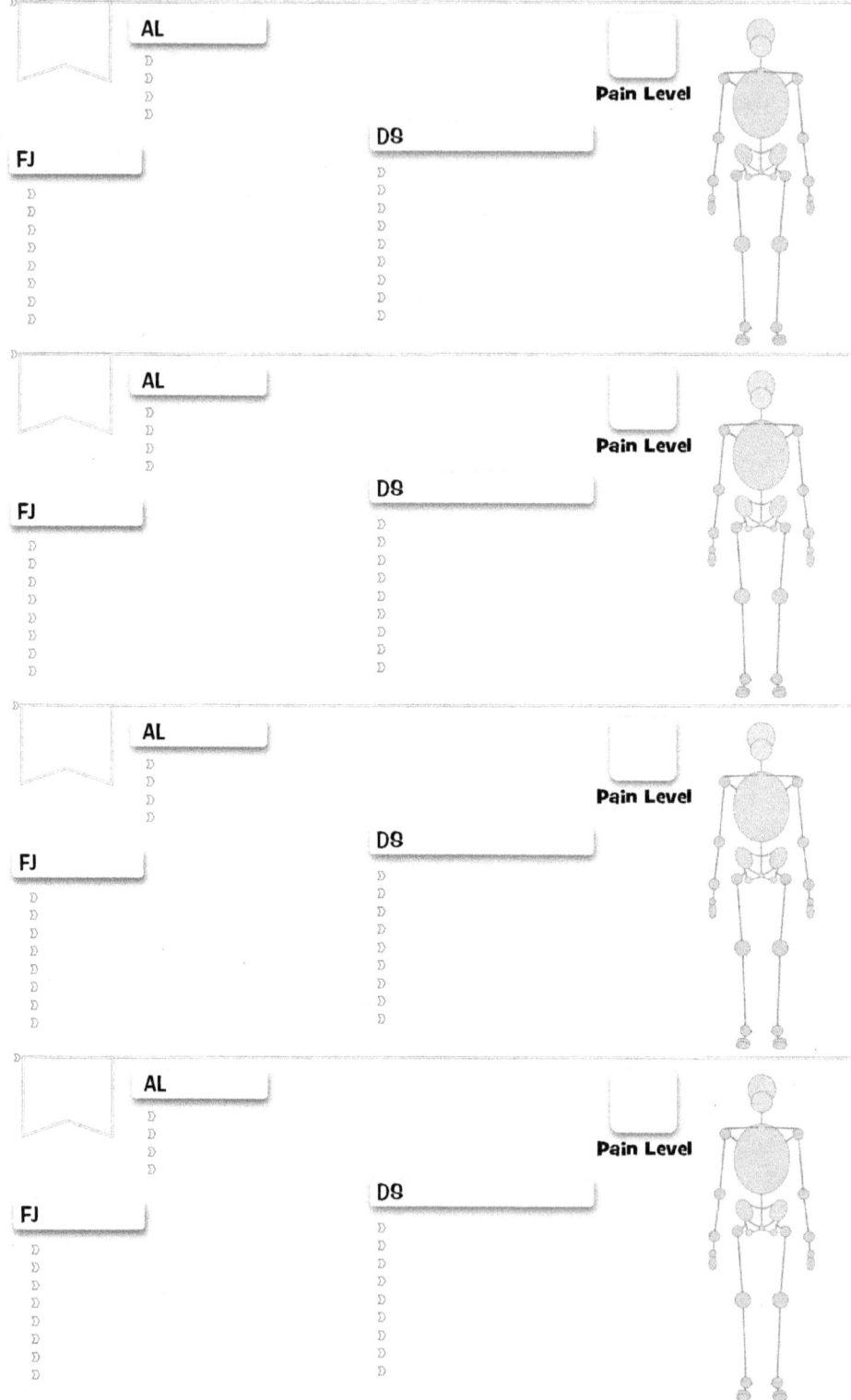

AL

FJ

DS

Pain Level

AL

FJ

DS

Pain Level

AL

FJ

DS

Pain Level

AL

FJ

DS

Pain Level

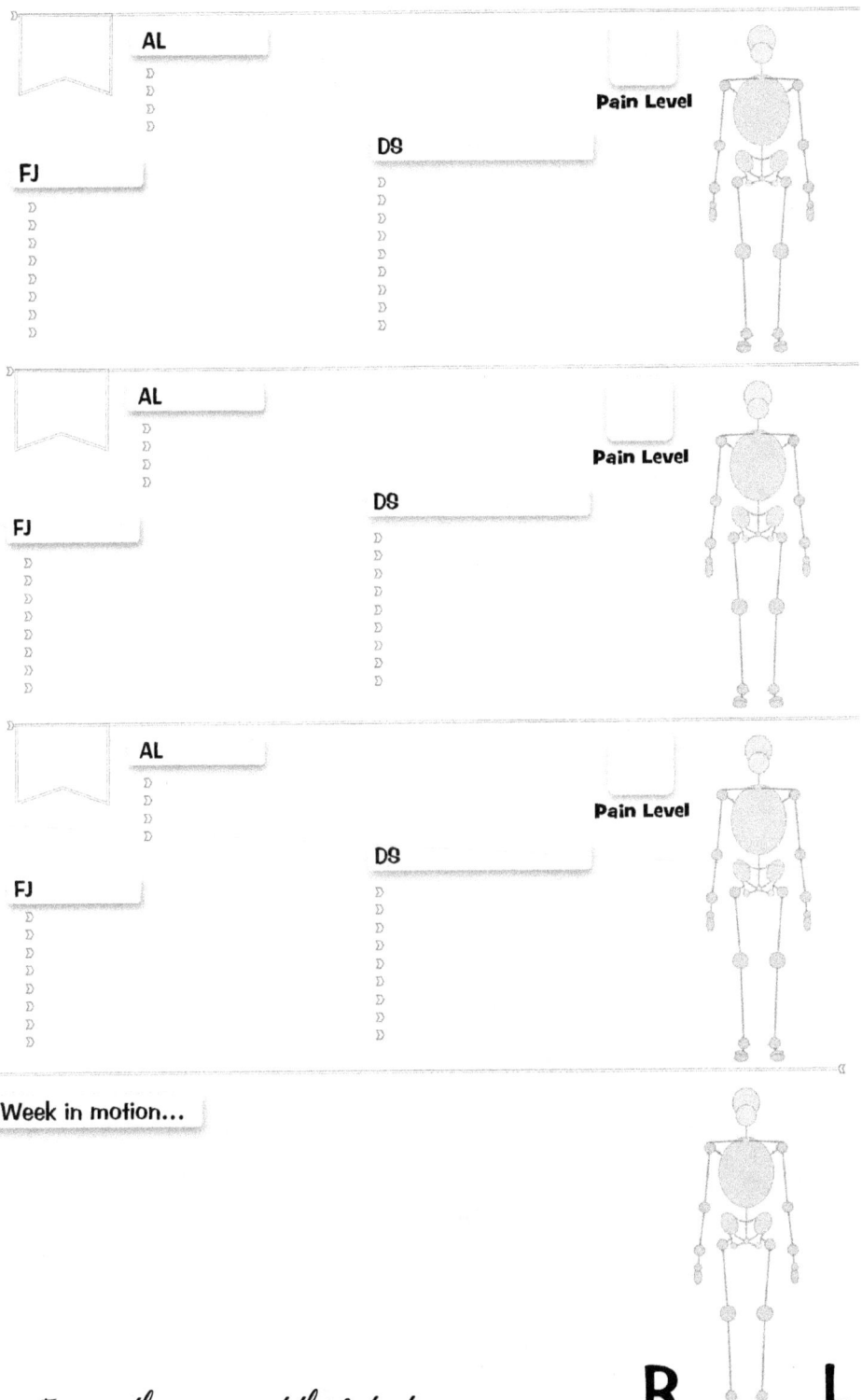

AL
- ⟩
- ⟩
- ⟩
- ⟩

Pain Level

FJ
- ⟩
- ⟩
- ⟩
- ⟩
- ⟩
- ⟩
- ⟩

DS
- ⟩
- ⟩
- ⟩
- ⟩
- ⟩
- ⟩
- ⟩

AL
- ⟩
- ⟩
- ⟩

Pain Level

FJ
- ⟩
- ⟩
- ⟩
- ⟩
- ⟩
- ⟩
- ⟩

DS
- ⟩
- ⟩
- ⟩
- ⟩
- ⟩
- ⟩
- ⟩

AL
- ⟩
- ⟩
- ⟩

Pain Level

FJ
- ⟩
- ⟩
- ⟩
- ⟩
- ⟩
- ⟩
- ⟩

DS
- ⟩
- ⟩
- ⟩
- ⟩
- ⟩
- ⟩
- ⟩

Week in motion...

Focus on the journey, not the destination. – UNK

R   L

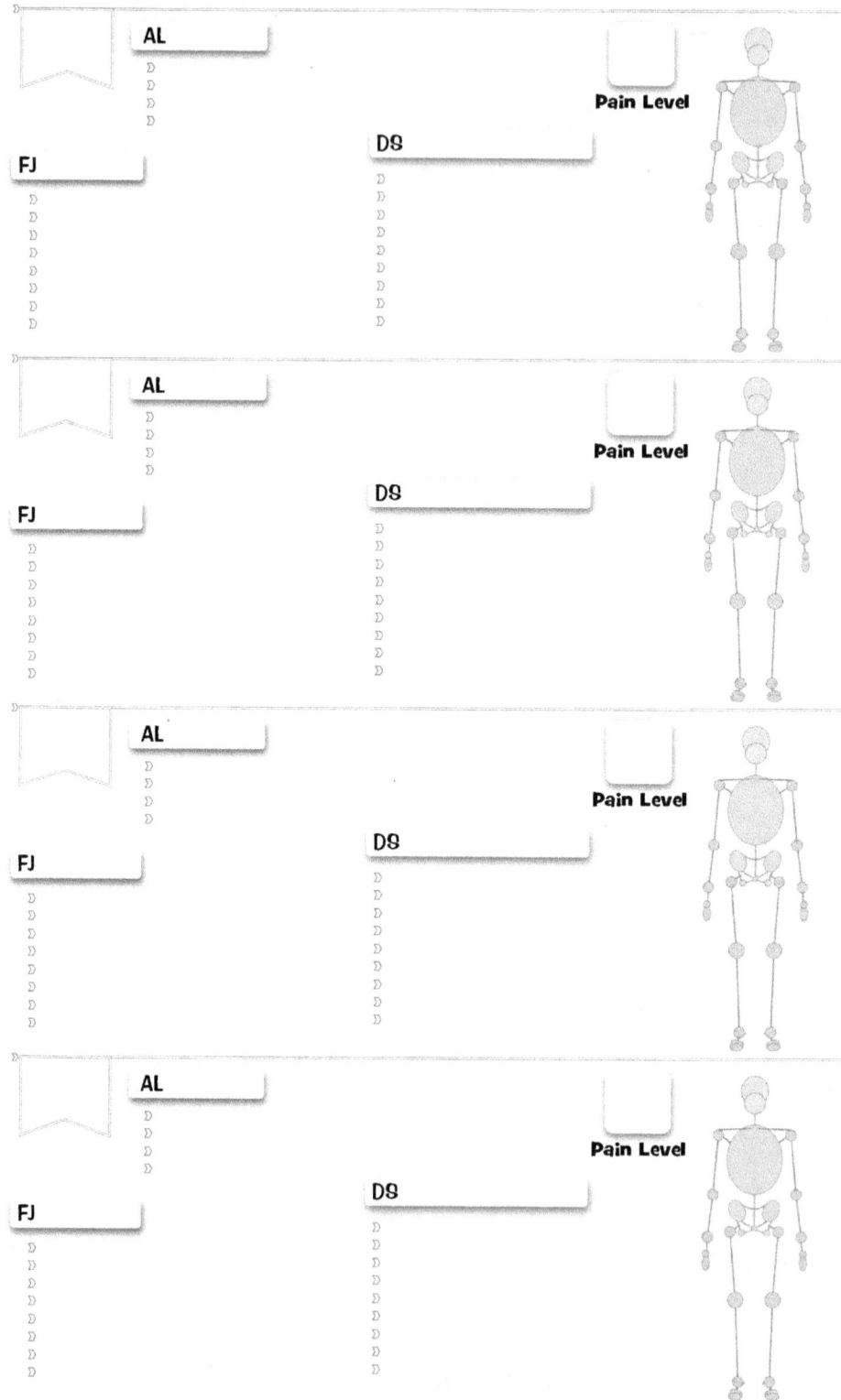

AL

FJ

DS

Pain Level

AL

FJ

DS

Pain Level

AL

FJ

DS

Pain Level

AL

FJ

DS

Pain Level

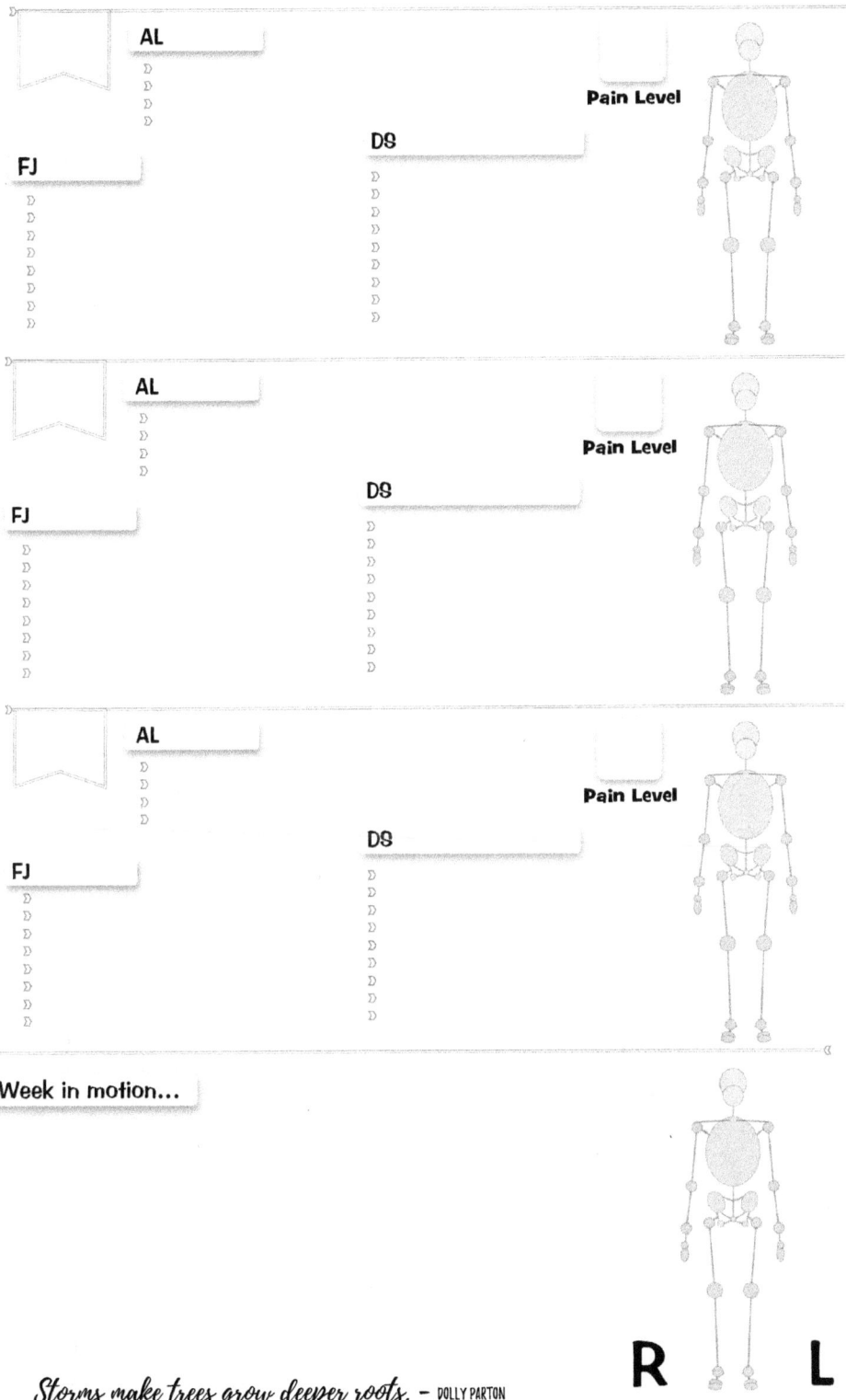

AL

FJ

DS

Pain Level

AL

FJ

DS

Pain Level

AL

FJ

DS

Pain Level

Week in motion...

R   L

Storms make trees grow deeper roots. — DOLLY PARTON

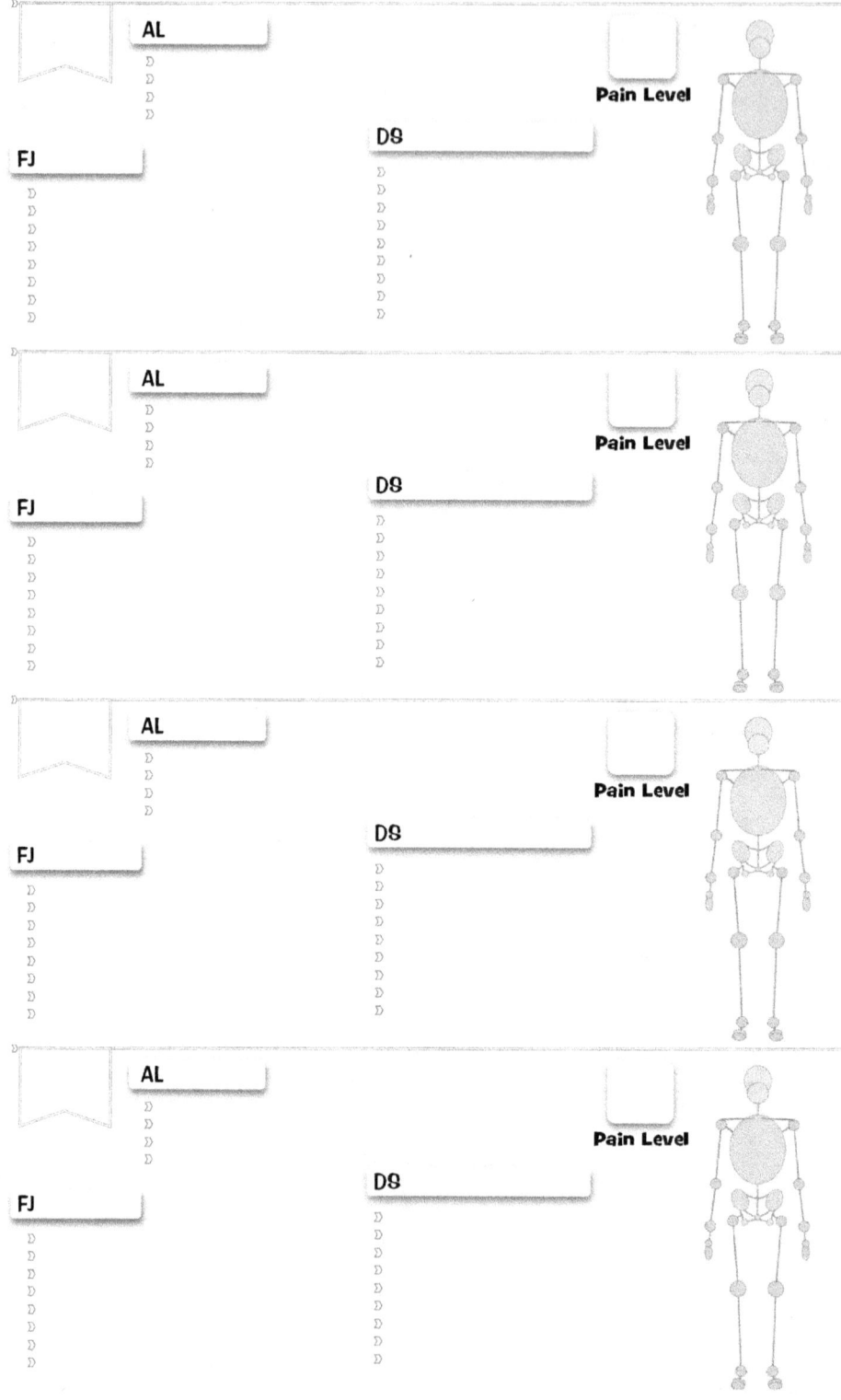

AL

FJ

Pain Level

DS

AL

FJ

Pain Level

DS

AL

FJ

Pain Level

DS

AL

FJ

Pain Level

DS

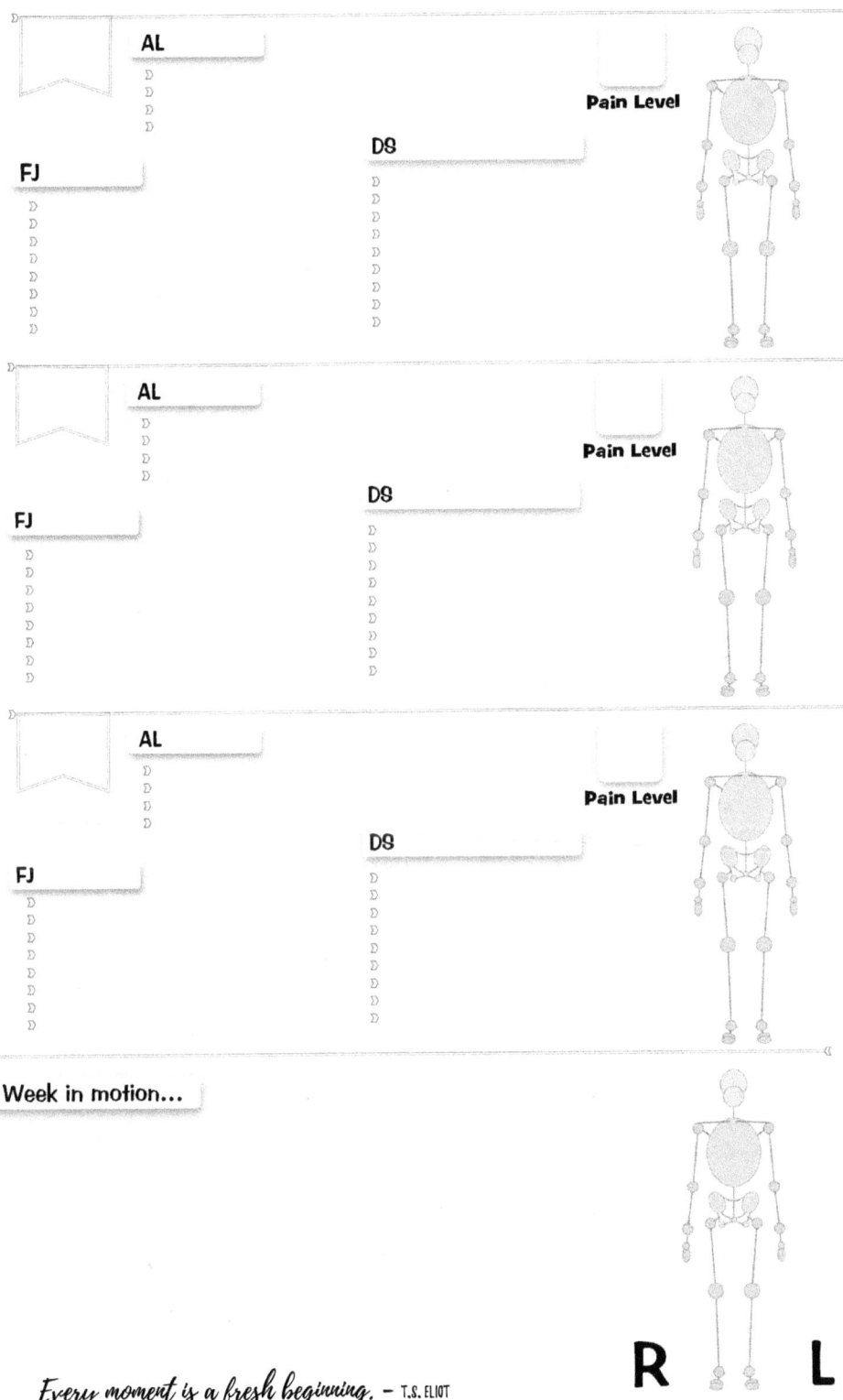

AL

Pain Level

FJ

DS

AL

Pain Level

FJ

DS

AL

Pain Level

FJ

DS

Week in motion...

R   L

Every moment is a fresh beginning. — T.S. ELIOT

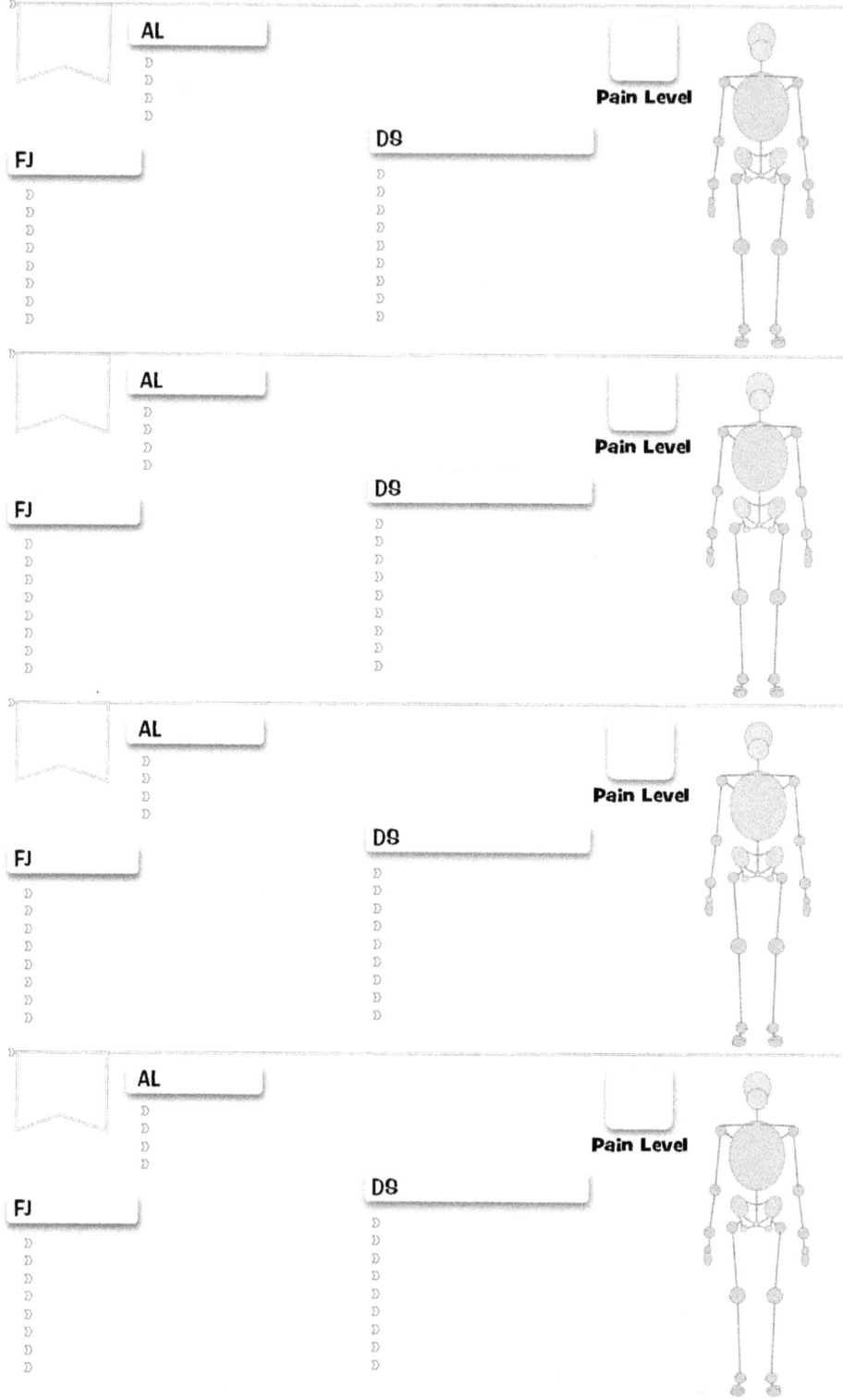

AL

FJ

Pain Level

DS

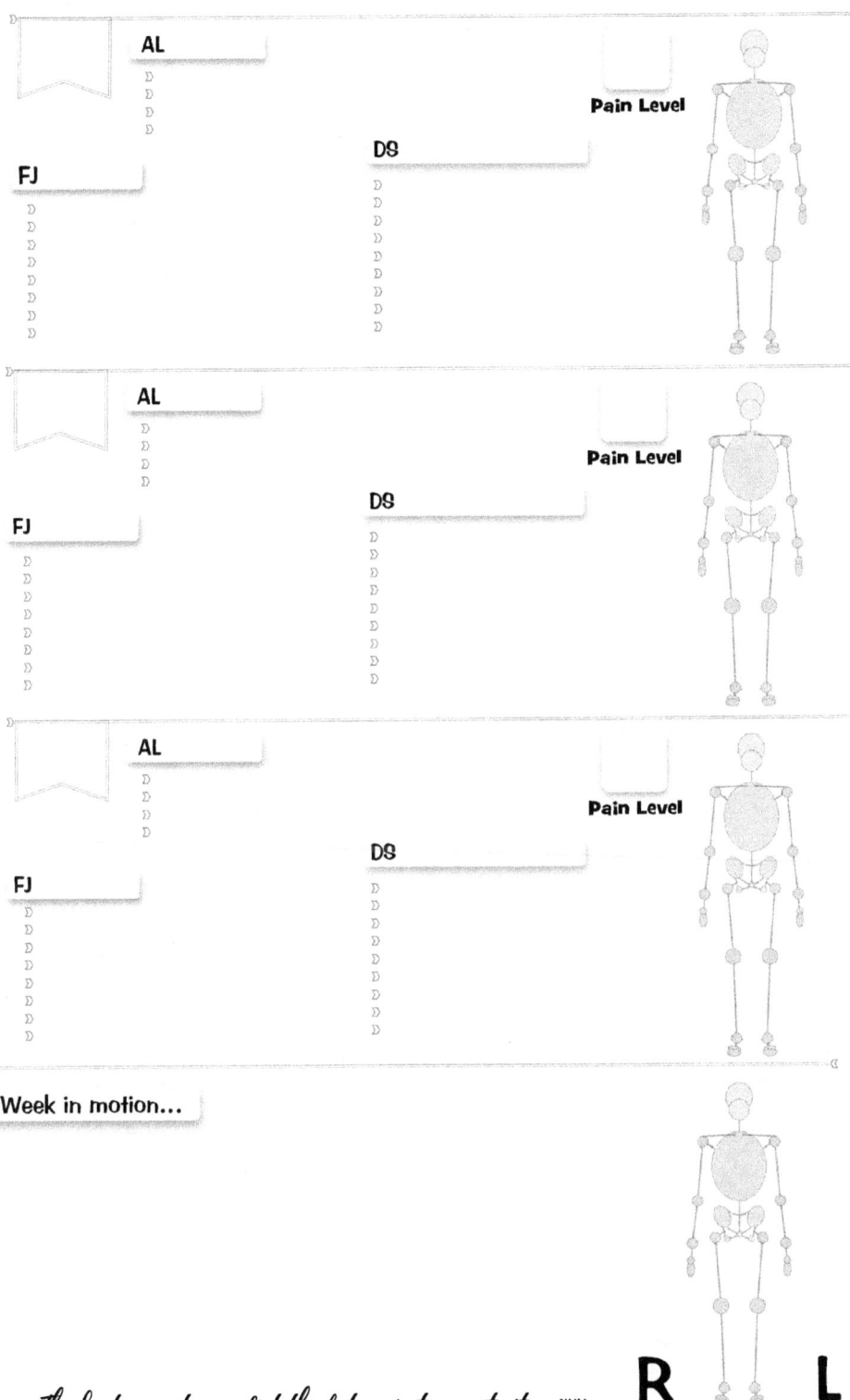

AL

FJ

DS

Pain Level

AL

FJ

DS

Pain Level

AL

FJ

DS

Pain Level

Week in motion...

R   **L**

The best way to predict the future is to create it. – UNK

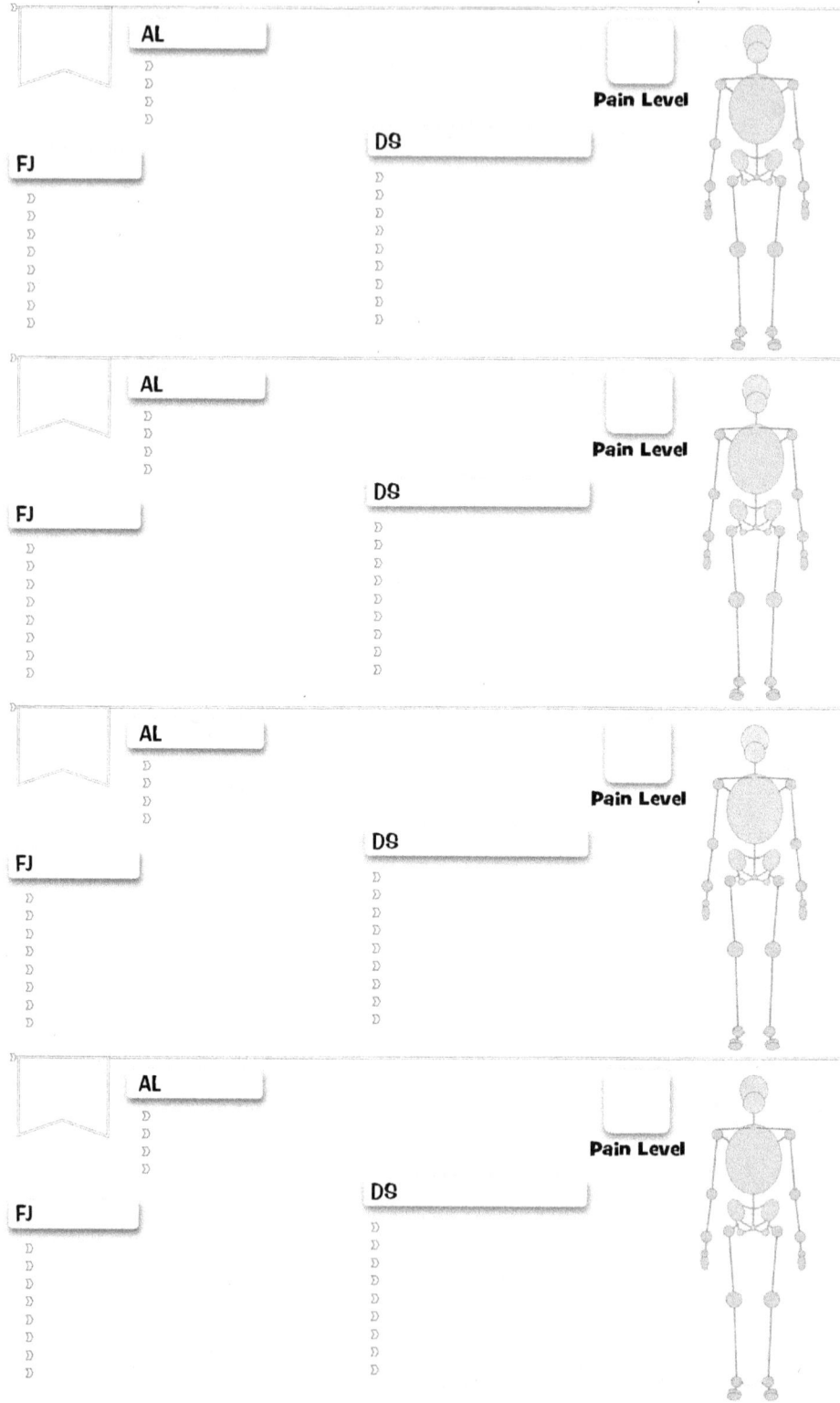

AL

FJ

DS

Pain Level

AL

- ⟩
- ⟩
- ⟩
- ⟩

Pain Level

FJ

- ⟩
- ⟩
- ⟩
- ⟩
- ⟩
- ⟩
- ⟩

DS

- ⟩
- ⟩
- ⟩
- ⟩
- ⟩
- ⟩
- ⟩

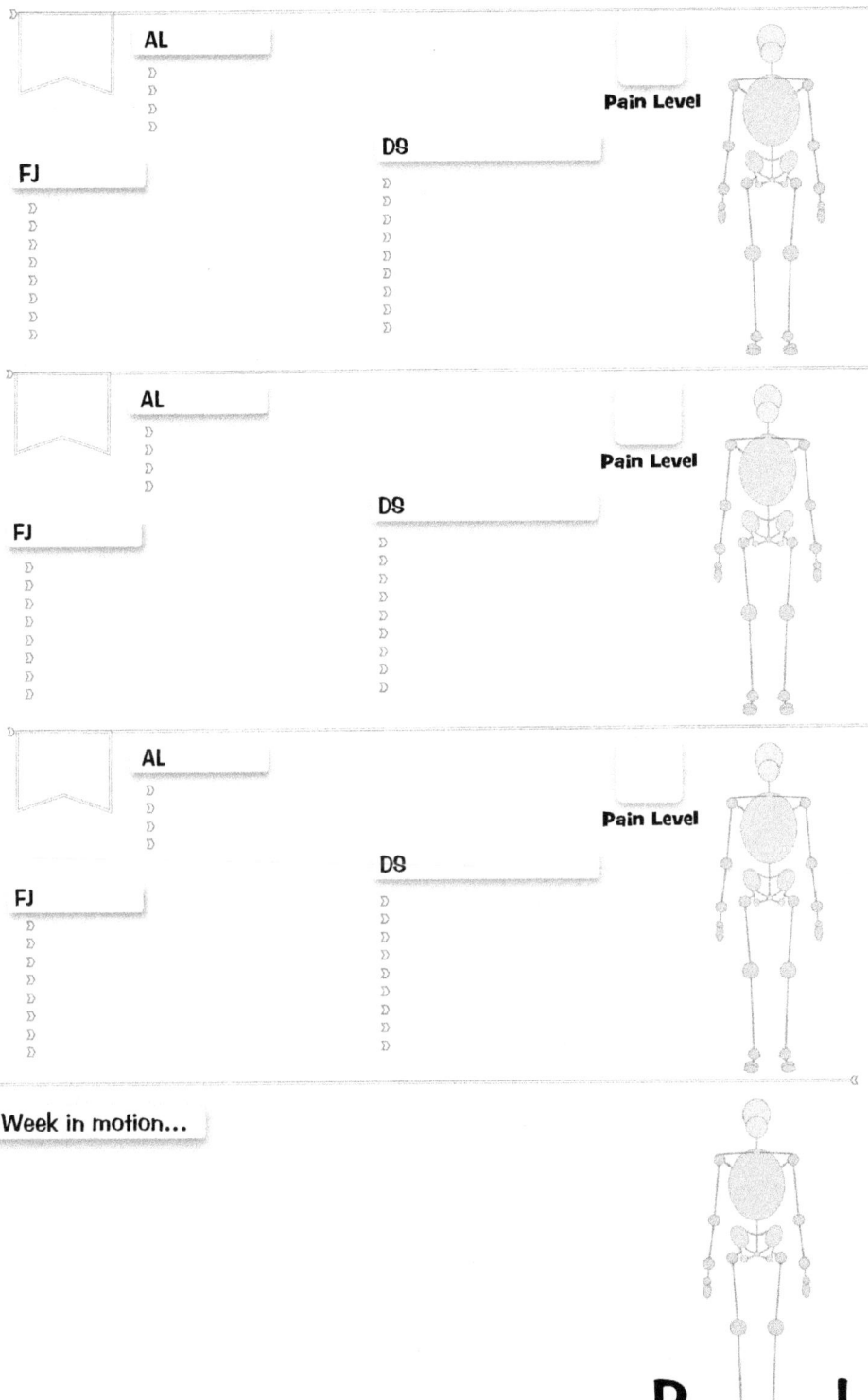

AL

- ⟩
- ⟩
- ⟩

Pain Level

FJ

- ⟩
- ⟩
- ⟩
- ⟩
- ⟩
- ⟩

DS

- ⟩
- ⟩
- ⟩
- ⟩
- ⟩
- ⟩

AL

- ⟩
- ⟩
- ⟩

Pain Level

FJ

- ⟩
- ⟩
- ⟩
- ⟩
- ⟩
- ⟩

DS

- ⟩
- ⟩
- ⟩
- ⟩
- ⟩
- ⟩

Week in motion...

R   **L**

Everything you want is on the other side of fear. – UNK

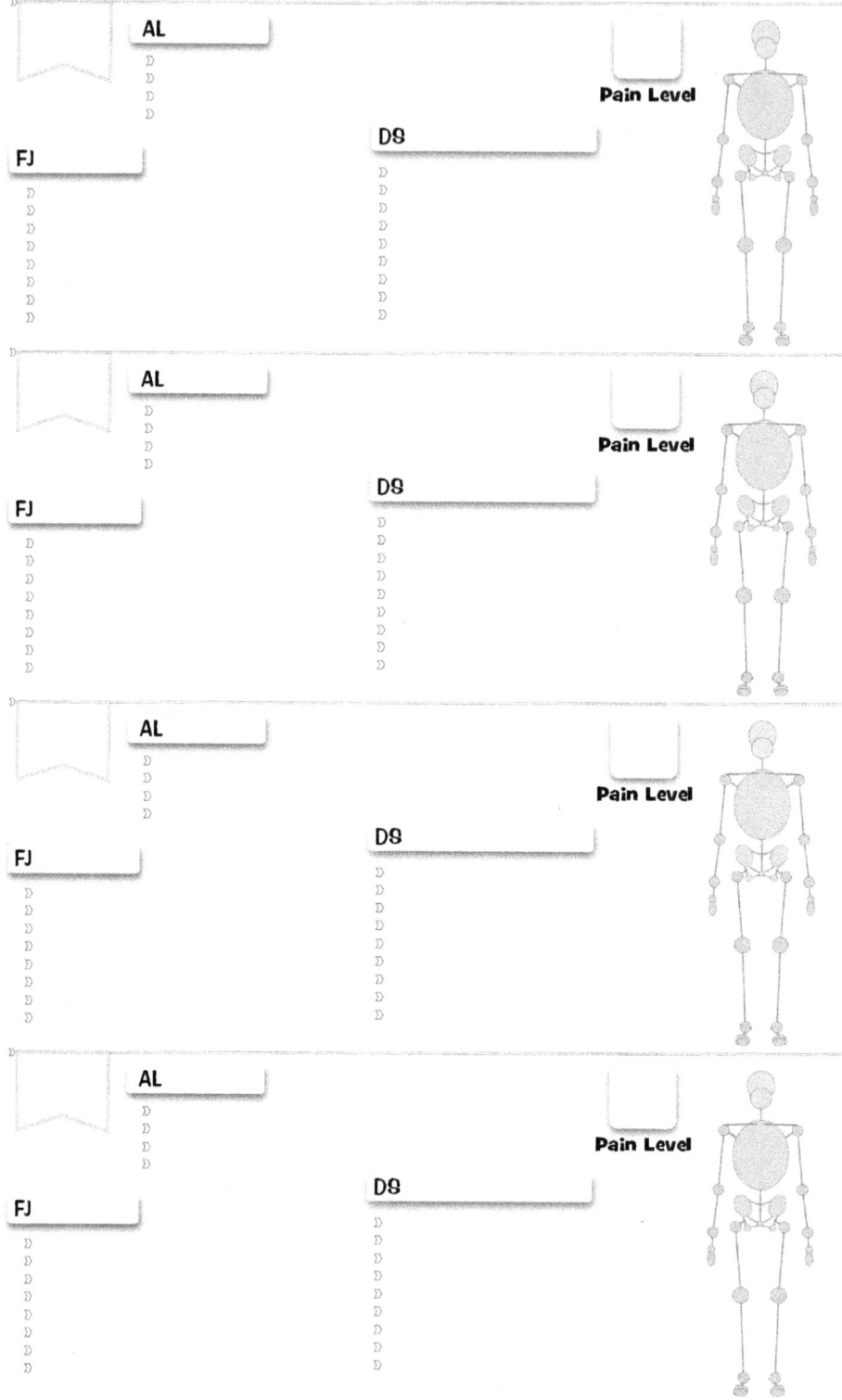

AL

FJ

DS

Pain Level

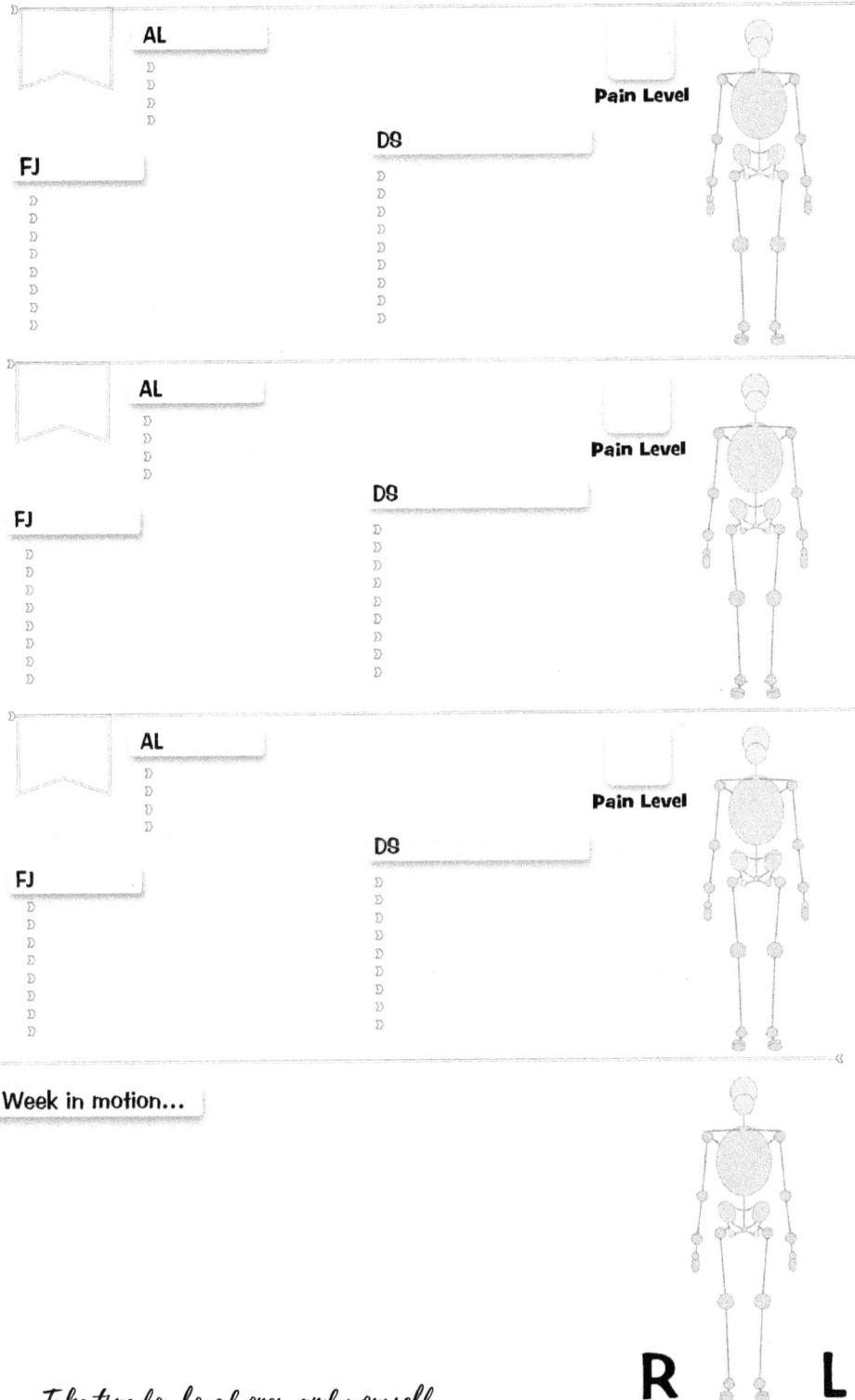

AL

Pain Level

FJ

DS

AL

Pain Level

FJ

DS

AL

Pain Level

FJ

DS

Week in motion...

Take time for loved ones, and yourself.

R   **L**

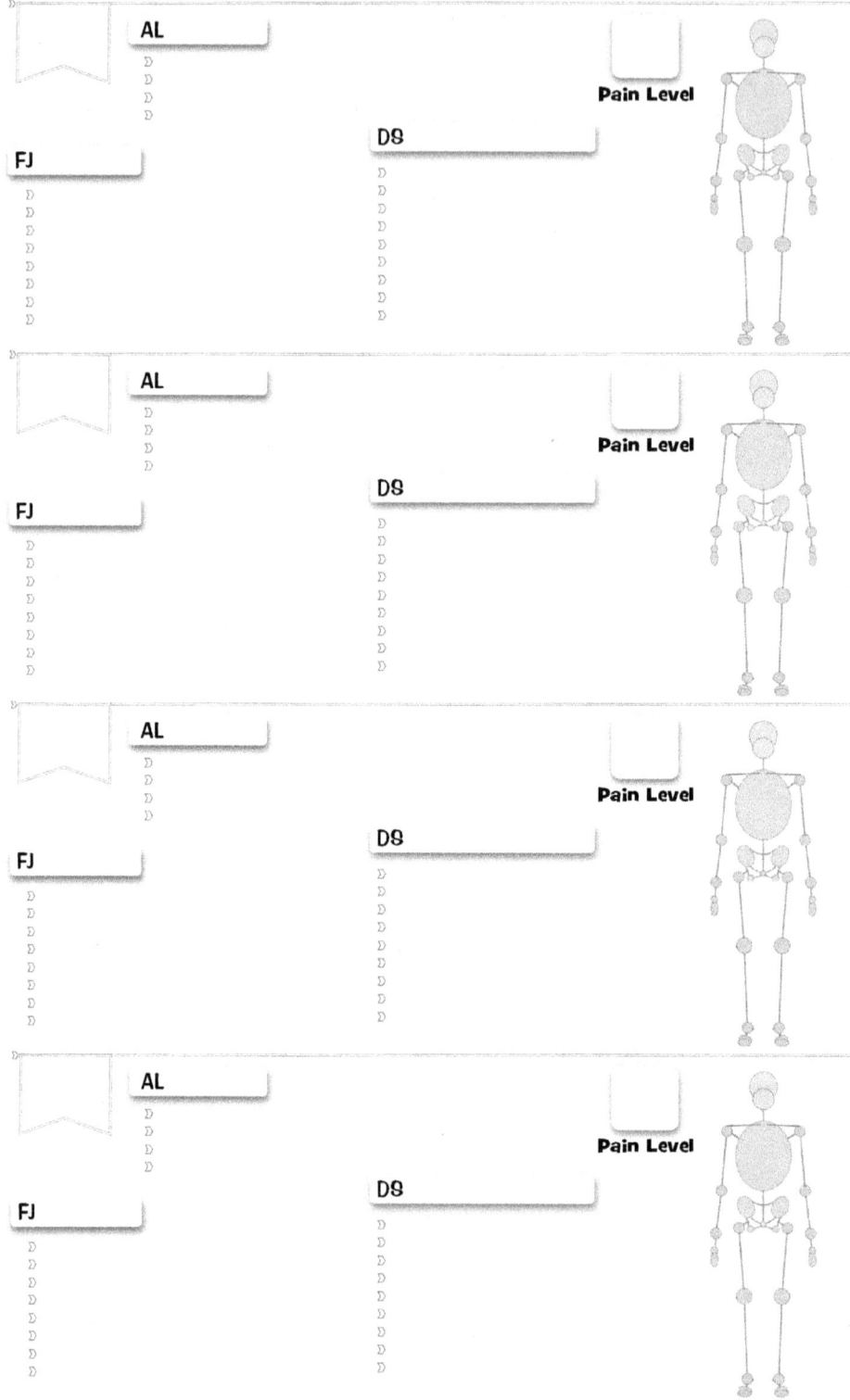

AL

FJ

DS

Pain Level

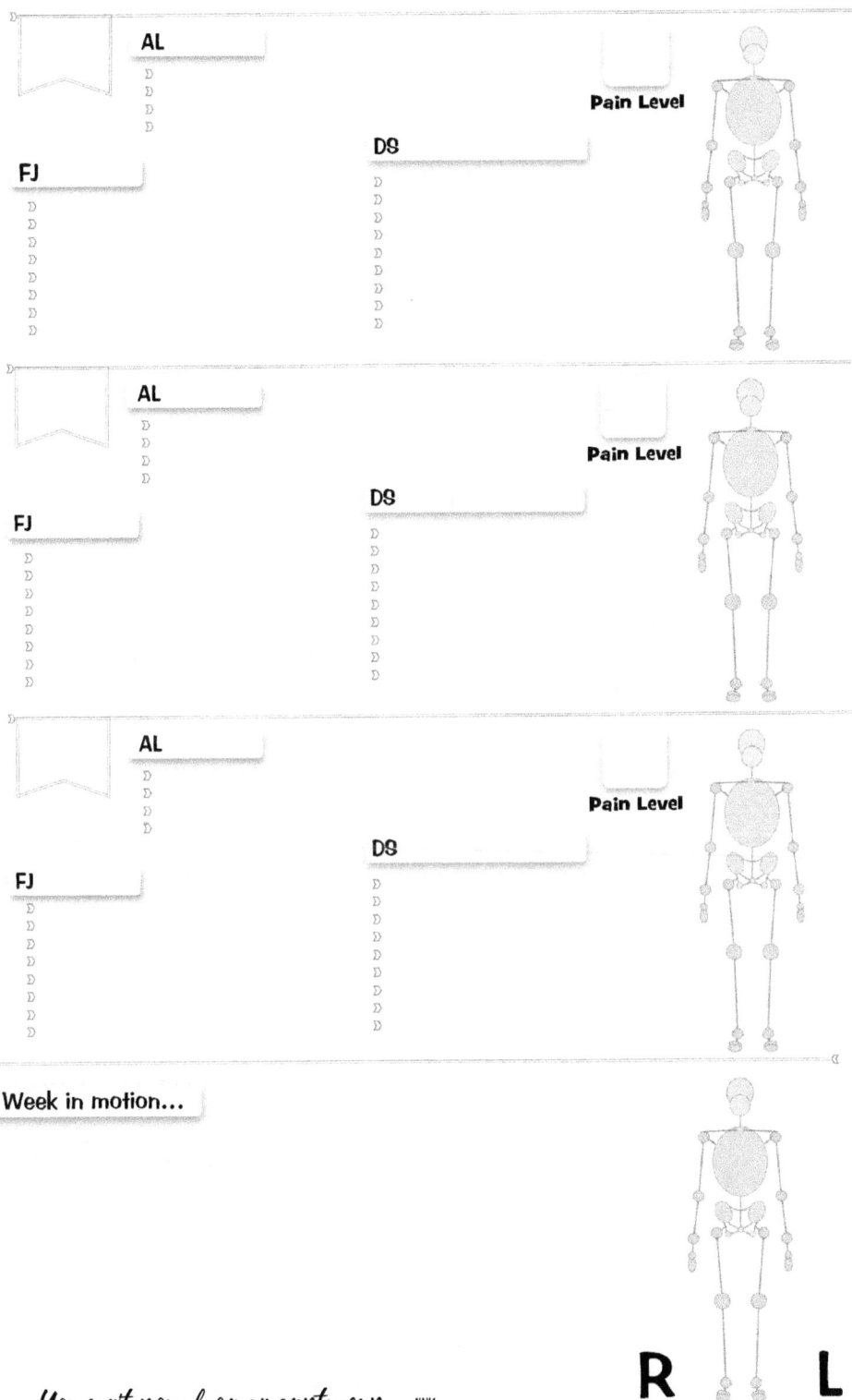

AL

FJ

DS

Pain Level

AL

Pain Level

FJ

DS

AL

Pain Level

DS

FJ

Week in motion...

R   L

You can't pour from an empty cup. - UNK

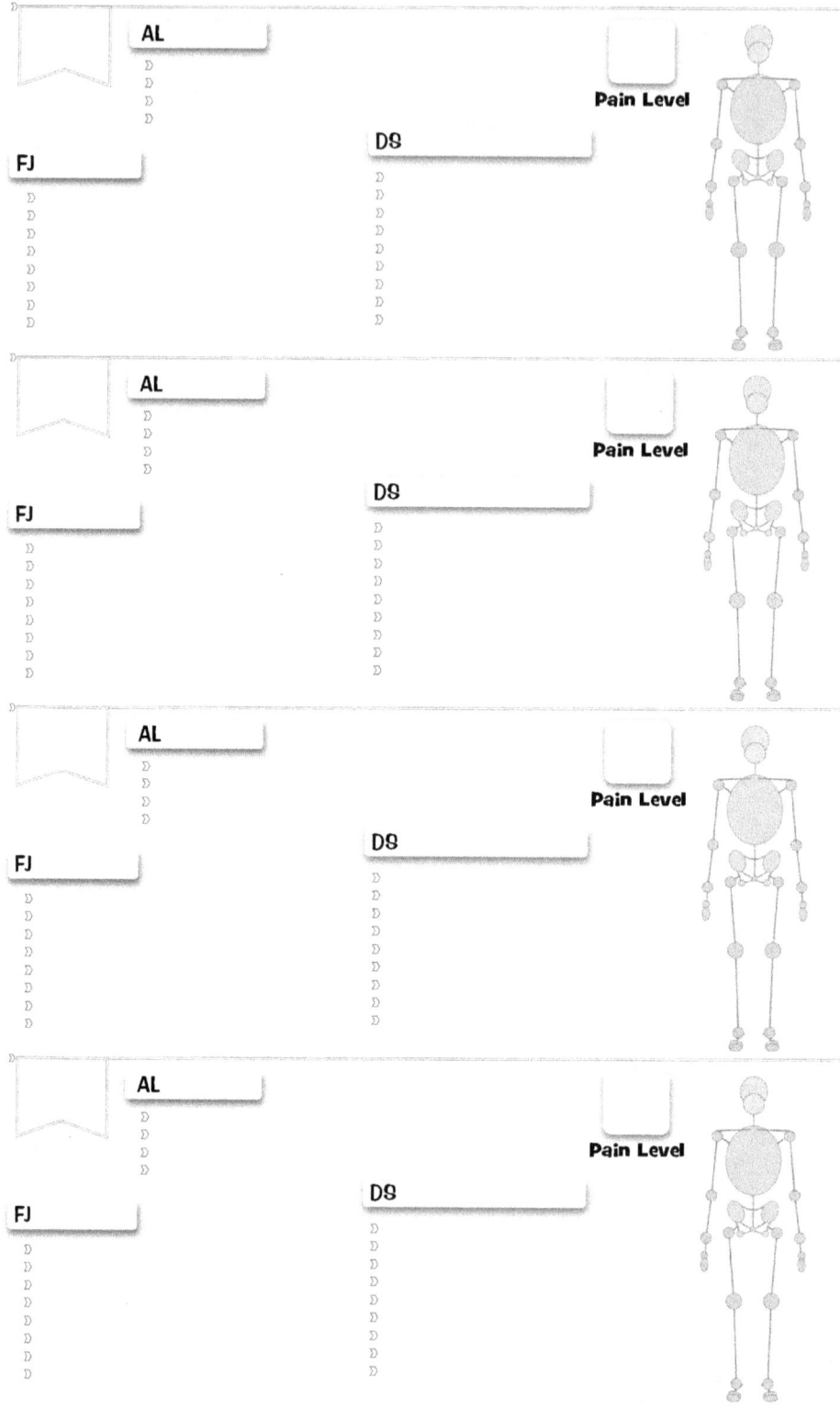

AL

FJ

DS

Pain Level

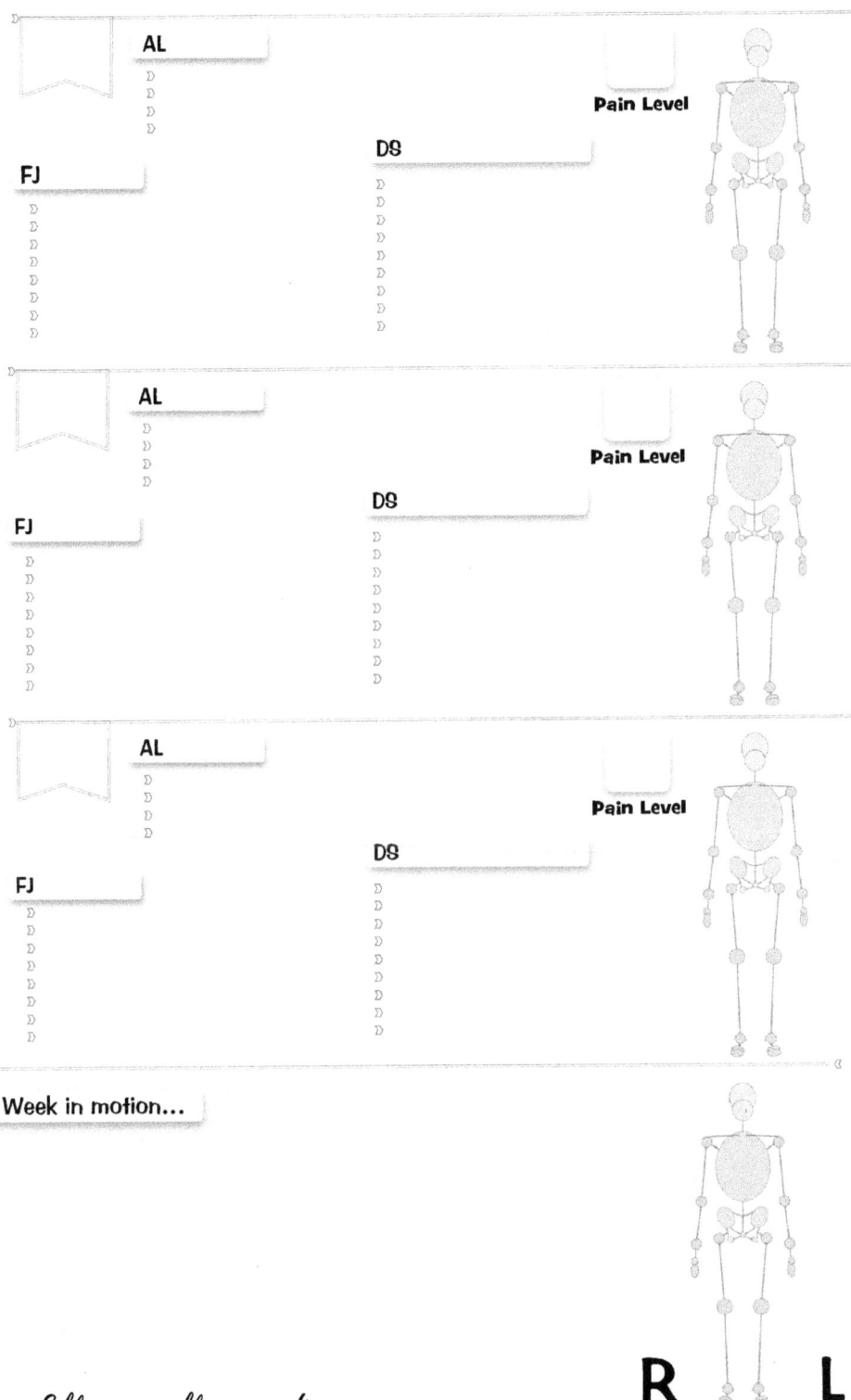

AL

Pain Level

FJ

DS

AL

Pain Level

FJ

DS

AL

Pain Level

FJ

DS

Week in motion...

Self care is self preservation.

R   **L**

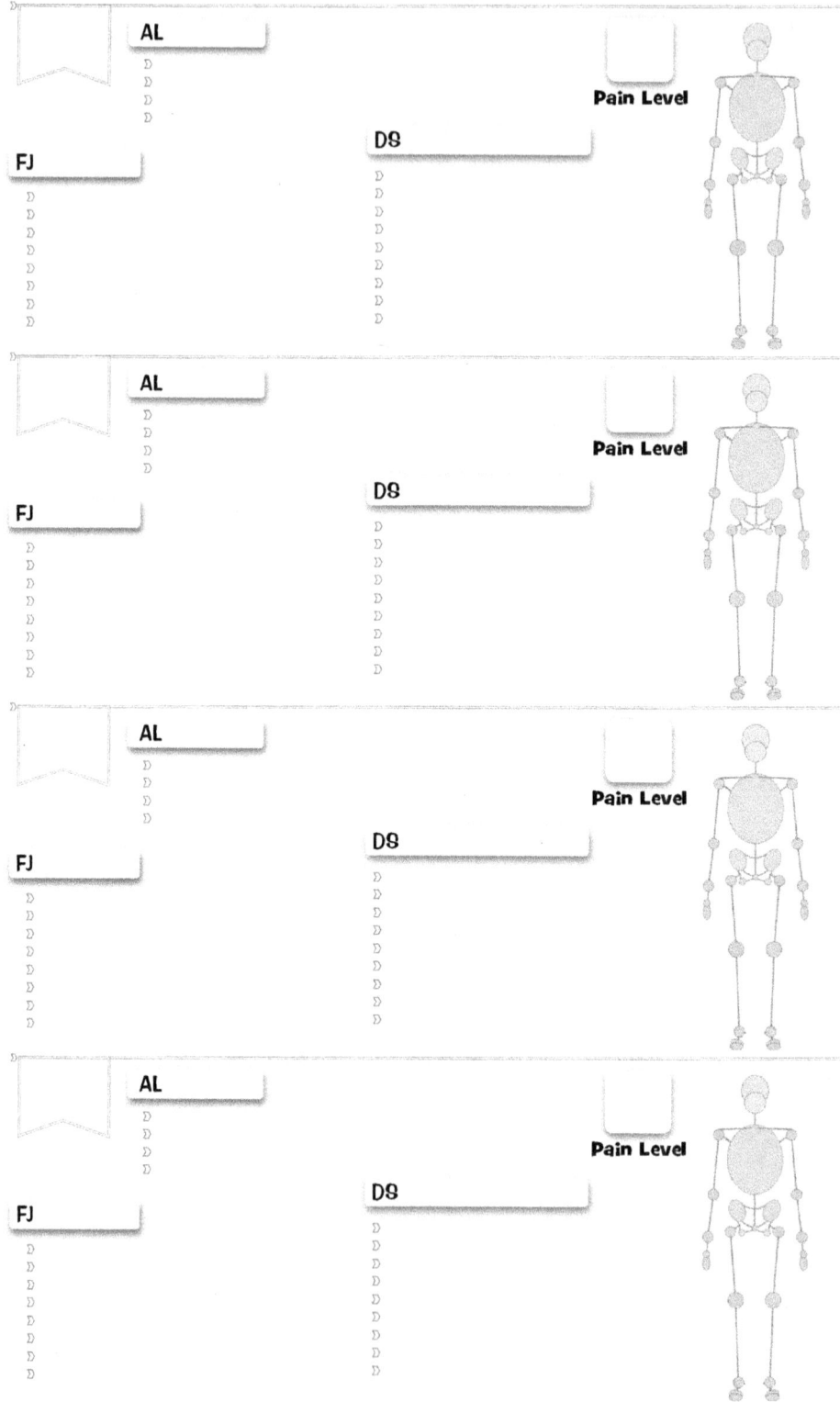

AL

FJ

DS

Pain Level

AL

FJ

DS

Pain Level

AL

FJ

DS

Pain Level

AL

FJ

DS

Pain Level

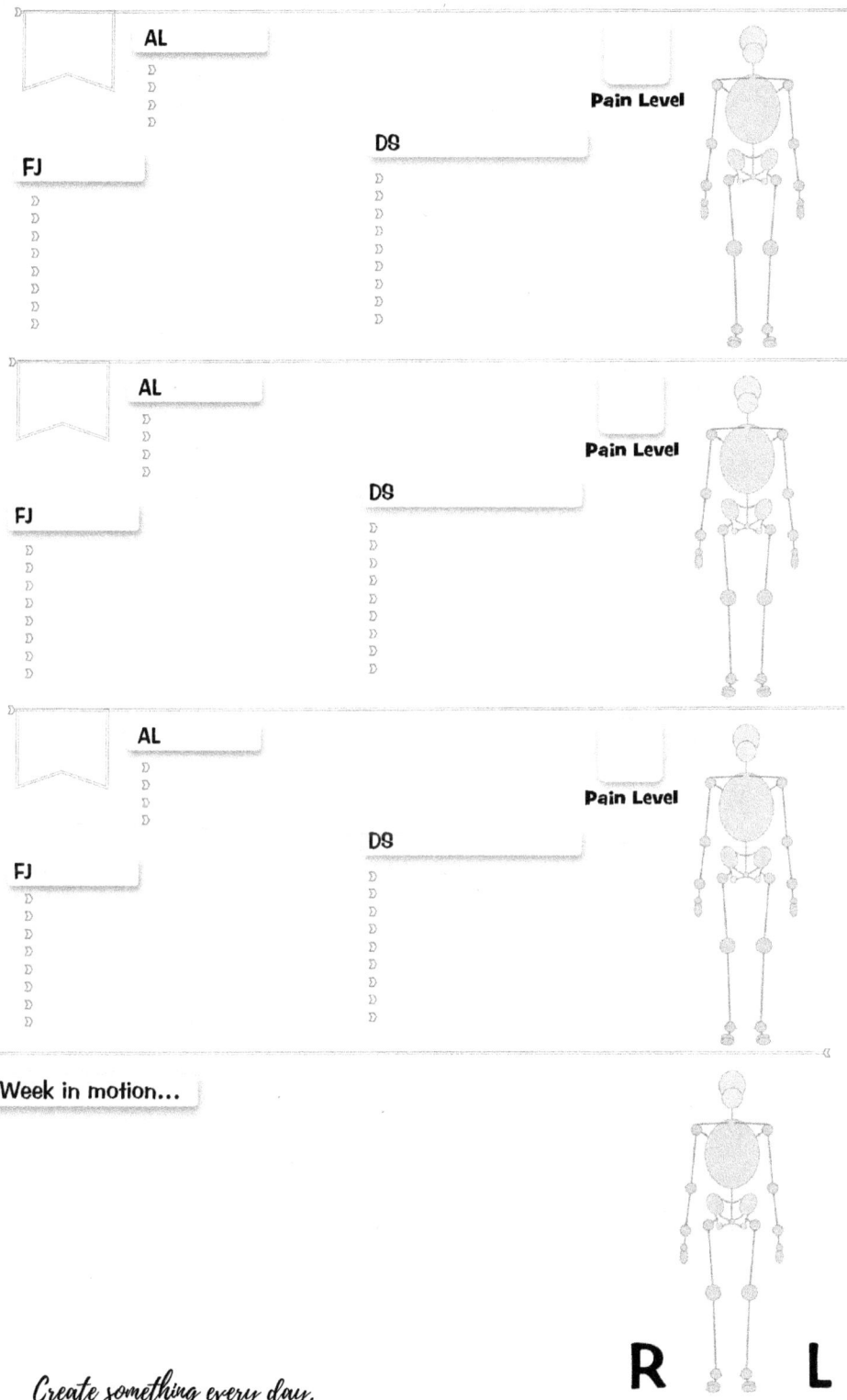

AL

Pain Level

FJ

DS

AL

Pain Level

FJ

DS

AL

Pain Level

FJ

DS

Week in motion...

Create something every day.

R   L

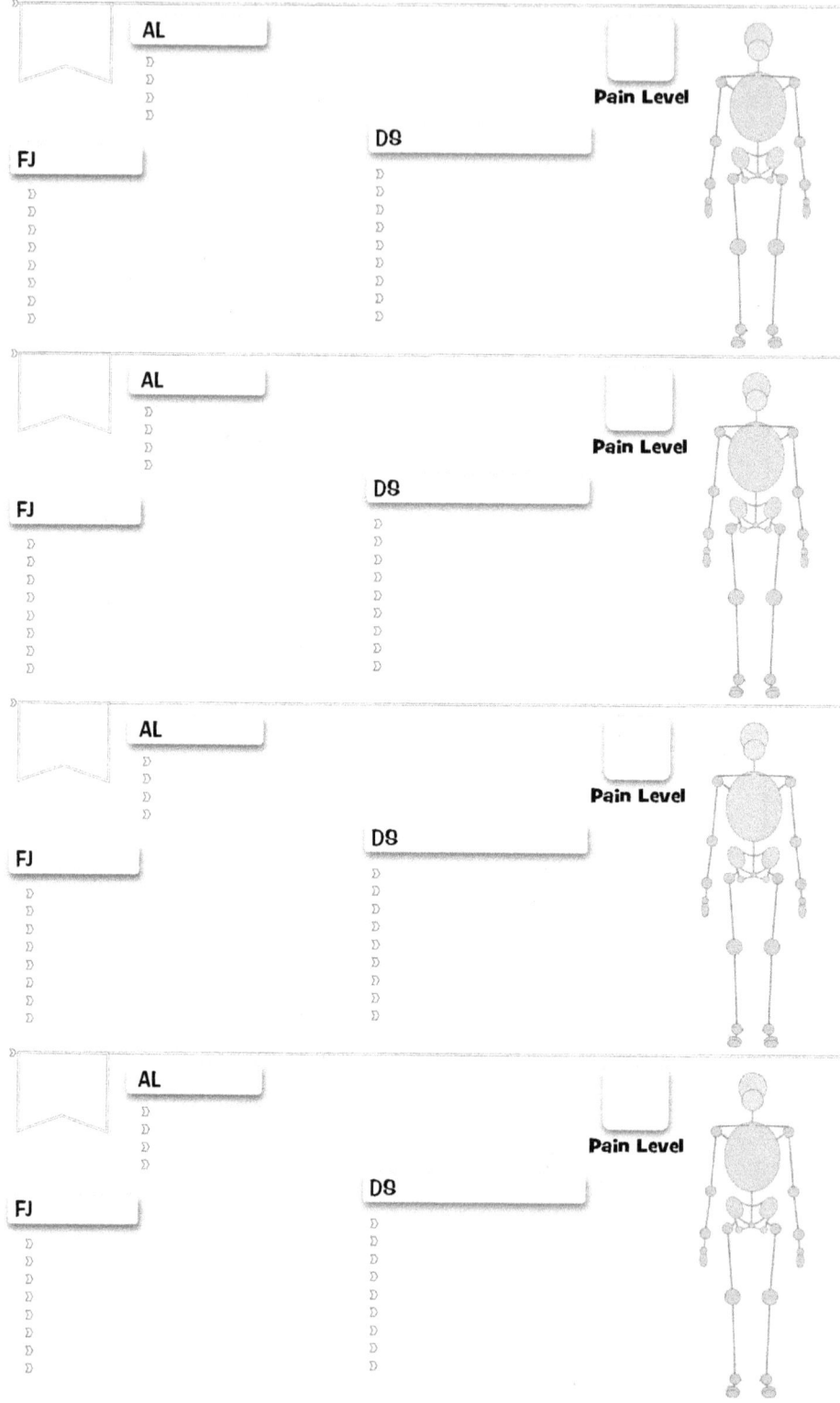

AL

FJ

DS

Pain Level

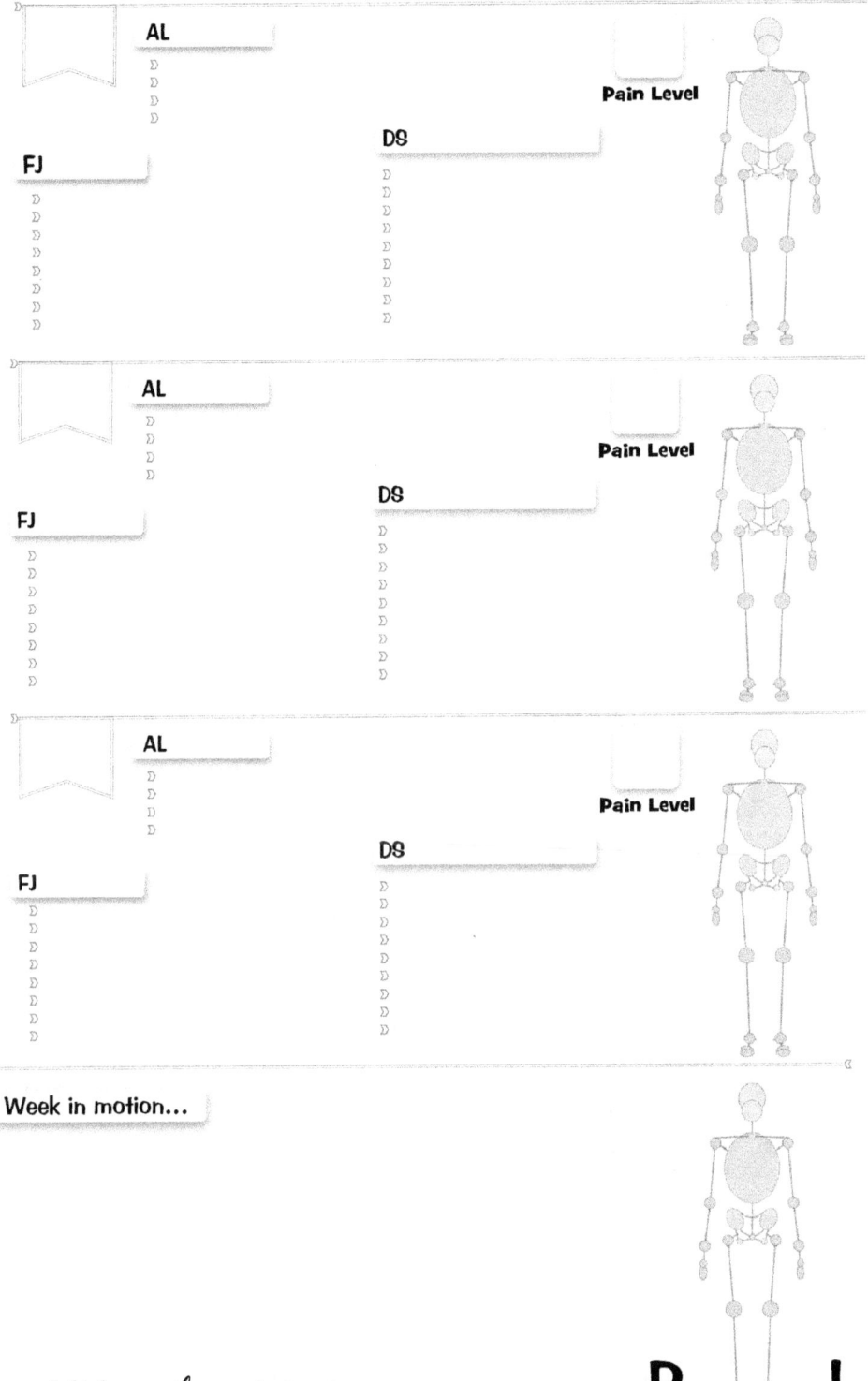

AL

- ⟩
- ⟩
- ⟩
- ⟩

Pain Level

FJ

- ⟩
- ⟩
- ⟩
- ⟩
- ⟩
- ⟩
- ⟩

DS

- ⟩
- ⟩
- ⟩
- ⟩
- ⟩
- ⟩
- ⟩

AL

- ⟩
- ⟩
- ⟩

Pain Level

FJ

- ⟩
- ⟩
- ⟩
- ⟩
- ⟩
- ⟩

DS

- ⟩
- ⟩
- ⟩
- ⟩
- ⟩
- ⟩
- ⟩

AL

- ⟩
- ⟩
- ⟩
- ⟩

Pain Level

FJ

- ⟩
- ⟩
- ⟩
- ⟩
- ⟩
- ⟩
- ⟩

DS

- ⟩
- ⟩
- ⟩
- ⟩
- ⟩
- ⟩
- ⟩

Week in motion...

Self love is the greatest medicine.

R   **L**

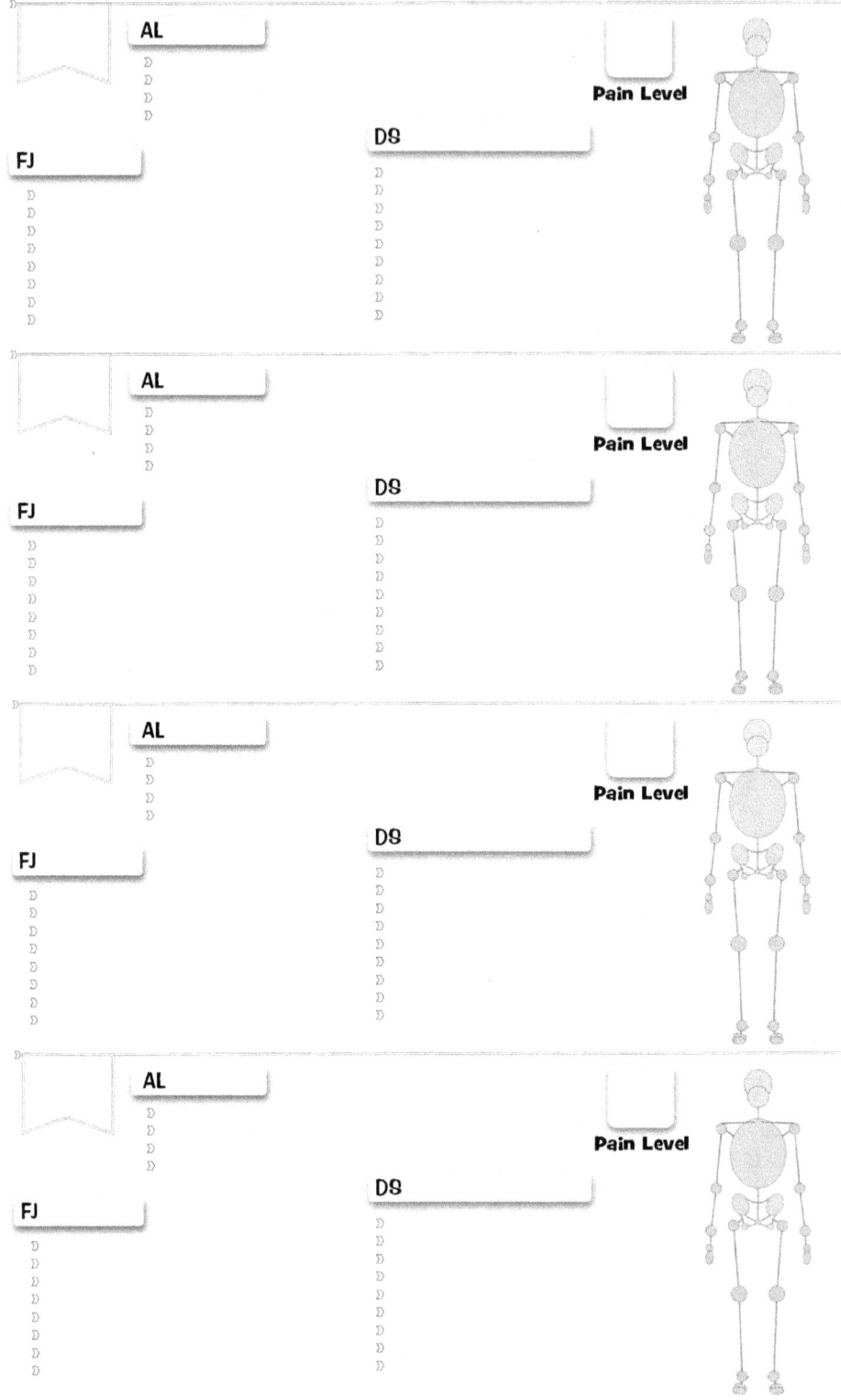

AL

FJ

DS

Pain Level

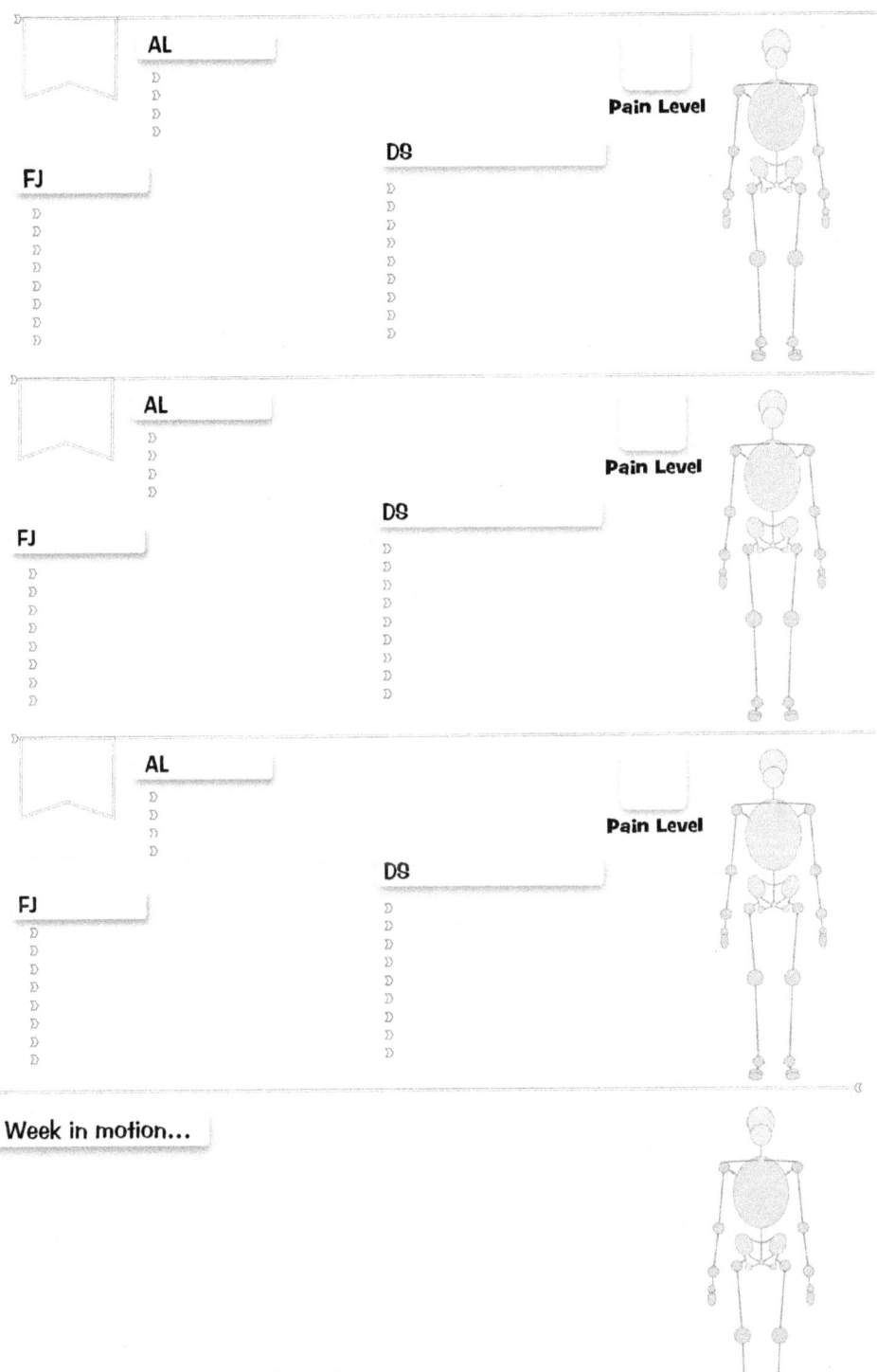

AL

FJ

DS

Pain Level

AL

FJ

DS

Pain Level

AL

FJ

DS

Pain Level

Week in motion...

Don't compare your life to others. There's no comparison between the sun and the moon. They shine when it's their time. – UNK

R **L**

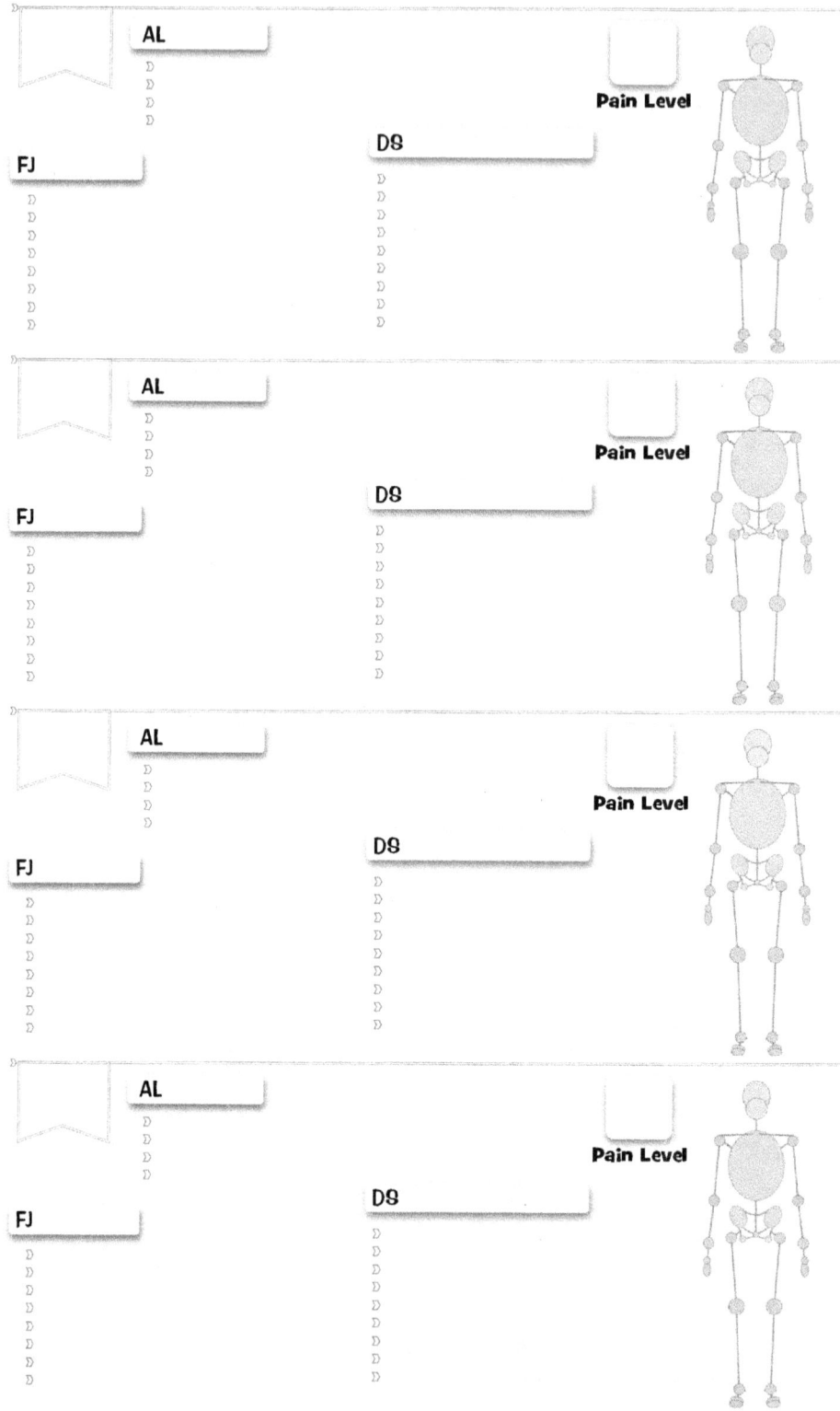

AL

FJ

DS

Pain Level

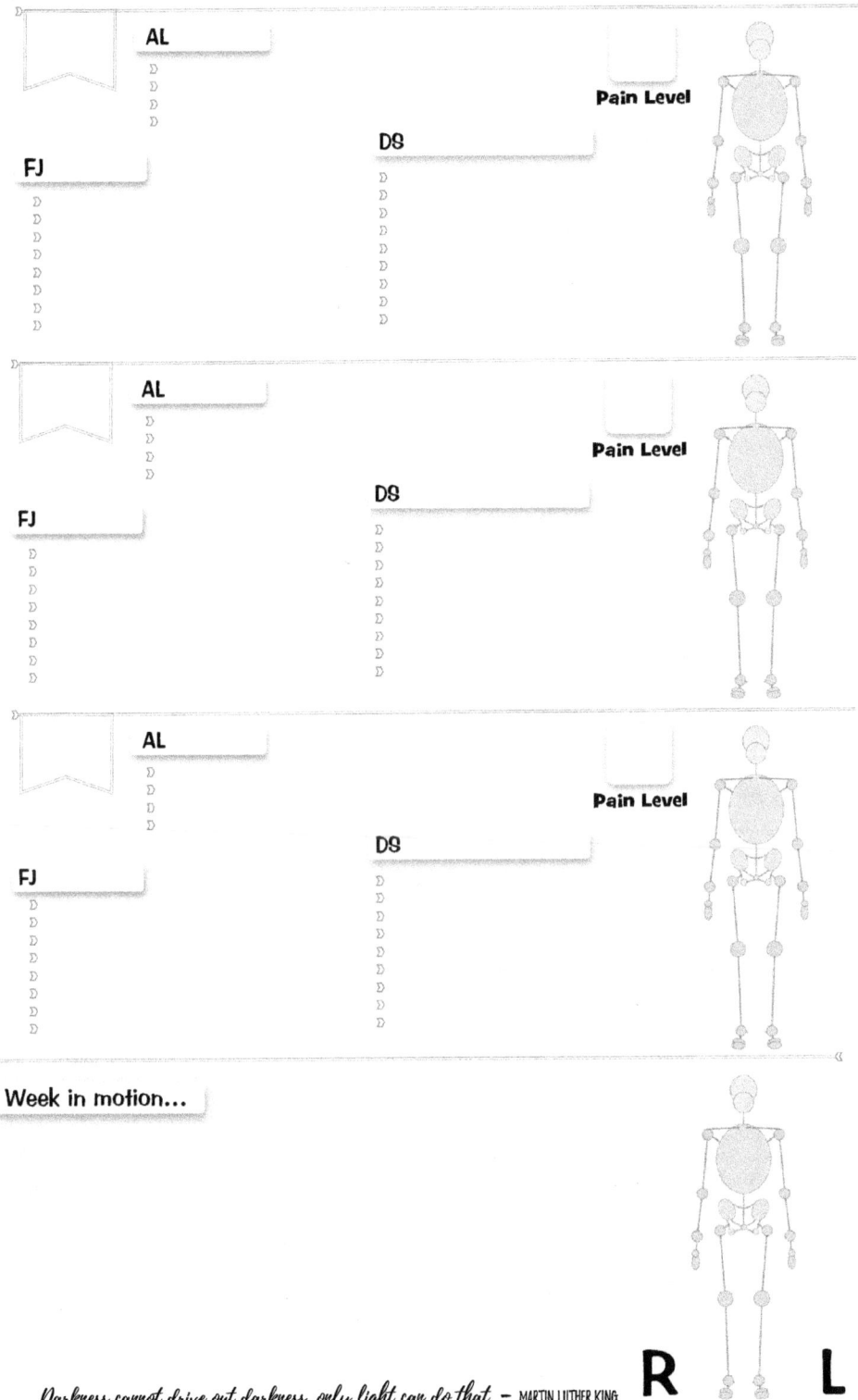

AL
D
D
D
D

FJ
D
D
D
D
D
D
D

DS
D
D
D
D
D
D
D
D

Pain Level

AL
D
D
D
D

FJ
D
D
D
D
D
D
D

DS
D
D
D
D
D
D
D

Pain Level

AL
D
D
D
D

FJ
D
D
D
D
D
D
D

DS
D
D
D
D
D
D
D

Pain Level

Week in motion...

Darkness cannot drive out darkness, only light can do that. — MARTIN LUTHER KING

R　**L**

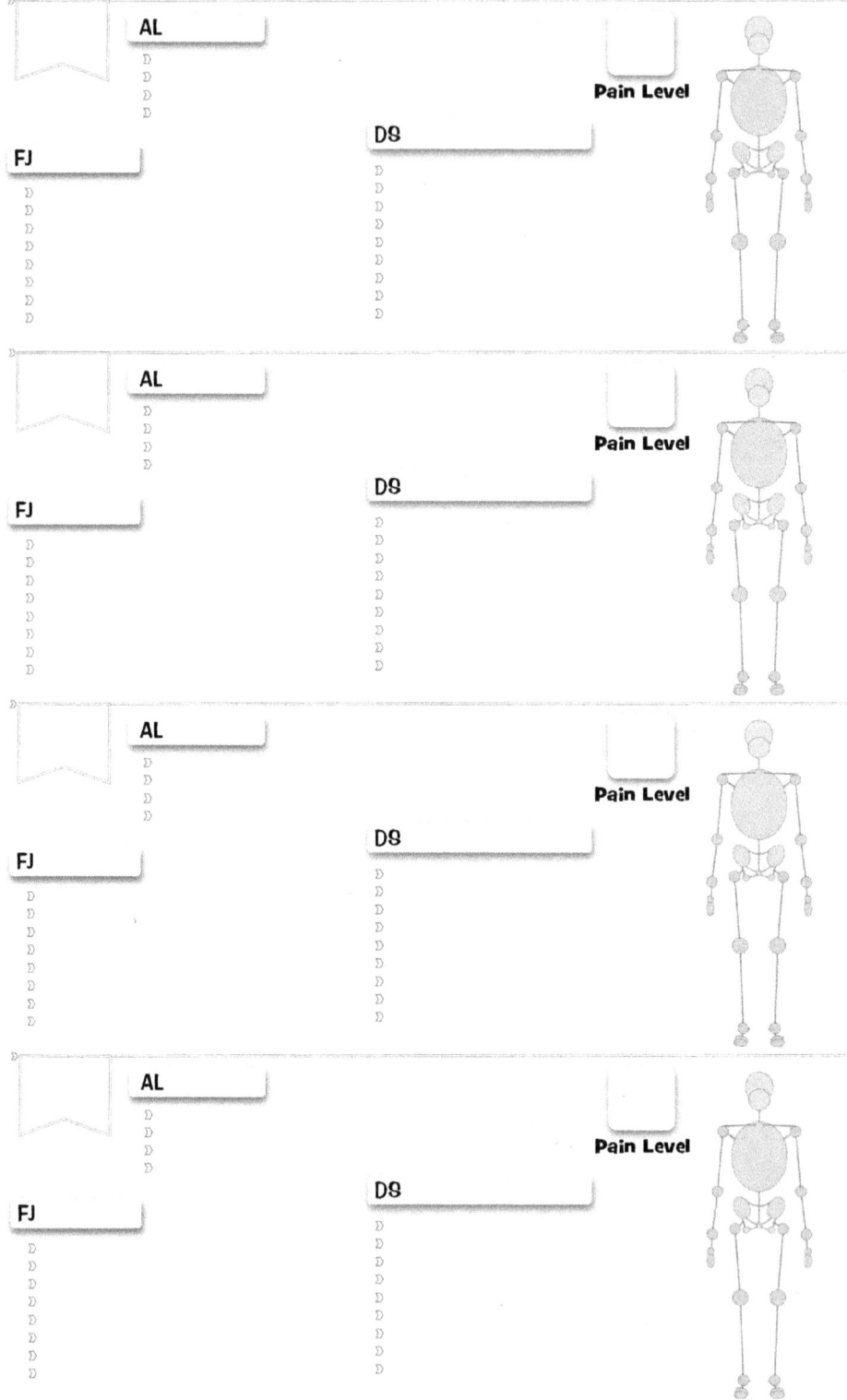

AL

FJ

DS

Pain Level

AL

FJ

DS

Pain Level

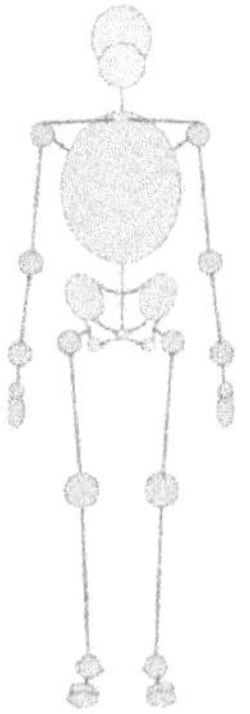

AL

FJ

DS

Pain Level

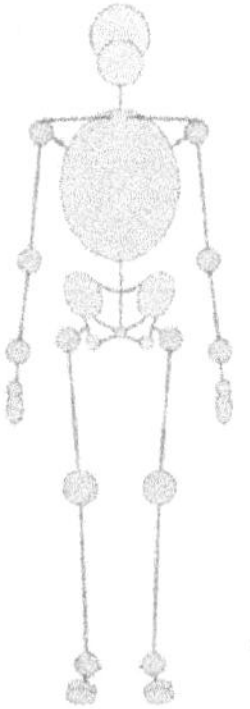

AL

FJ

DS

Pain Level

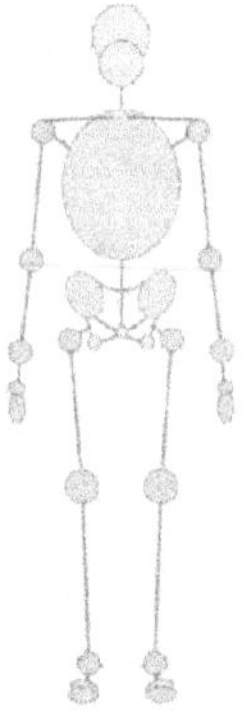

Week in motion...

Just because things aren't going the way you planned doesn't mean they aren't going the way they should. – UNK

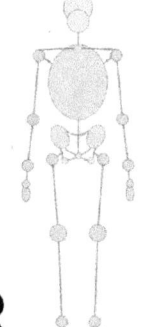

R   **L**

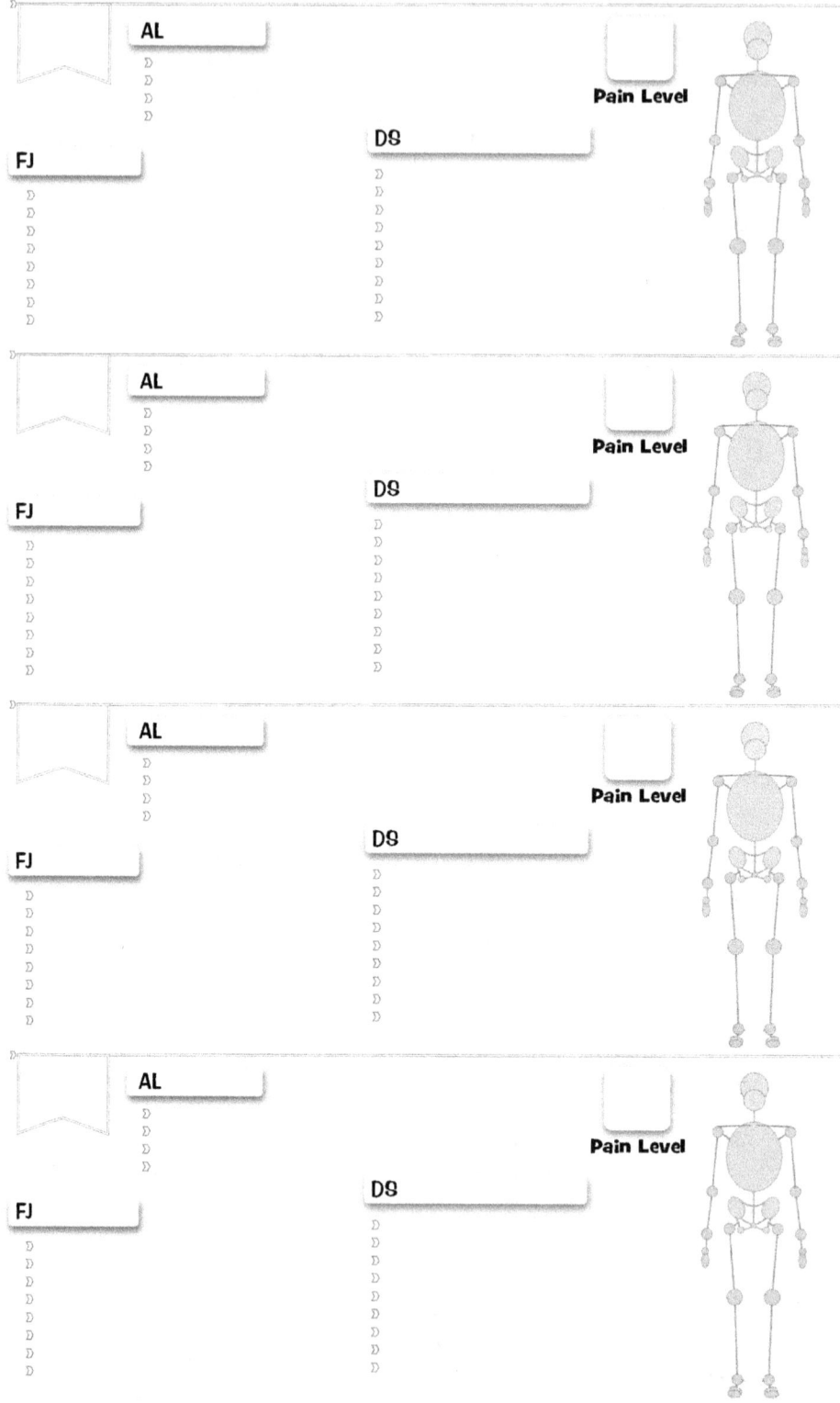

AL

FJ

DS

Pain Level

AL

FJ

DS

Pain Level

AL

FJ

DS

Pain Level

AL

FJ

DS

Pain Level

AL

〉
〉
〉
〉

FJ

〉
〉
〉
〉
〉
〉
〉

DS

〉
〉
〉
〉
〉
〉

Pain Level

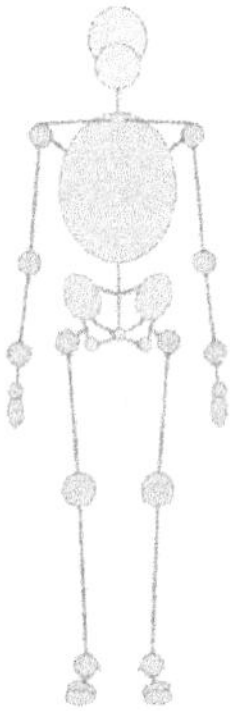

AL

〉
〉
〉
〉

FJ

〉
〉
〉
〉
〉
〉
〉

DS

〉
〉
〉
〉
〉
〉
〉

Pain Level

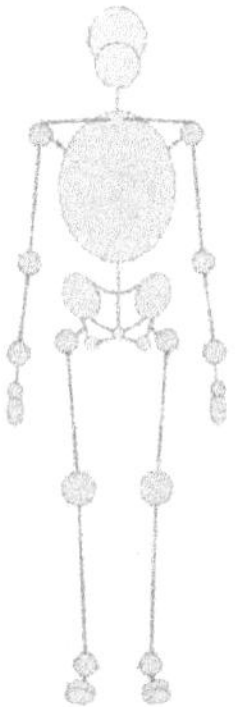

AL

〉
〉
〉
〉

FJ

〉
〉
〉
〉
〉
〉
〉

DS

〉
〉
〉
〉
〉
〉
〉

Pain Level

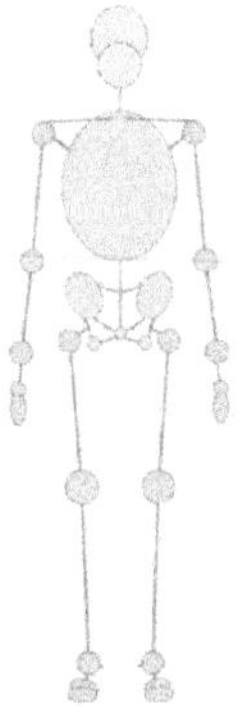

Week in motion...

When you make a commitment to yourself, the most important part is showing up.

R   L

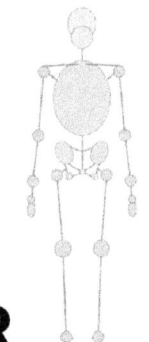

AL
  ))
  ))
  ))
  ))

FJ
  ))
  ))
  ))
  ))
  ))
  ))
  ))

DS
  ))
  ))
  ))
  ))
  ))
  ))
  ))

Pain Level

AL
  ))
  ))
  ))
  ))

FJ
  ))
  ))
  ))
  ))
  ))
  ))

DS
  ))
  ))
  ))
  ))
  ))
  ))
  ))

Pain Level

AL
  ))
  ))
  ))

FJ
  ))
  ))
  ))
  ))
  ))
  ))

DS
  ))
  ))
  ))
  ))
  ))
  ))

Pain Level

AL
  ))
  ))
  ))
  ))

FJ
  ))
  ))
  ))
  ))
  ))
  ))

DS
  ))
  ))
  ))
  ))
  ))
  ))

Pain Level

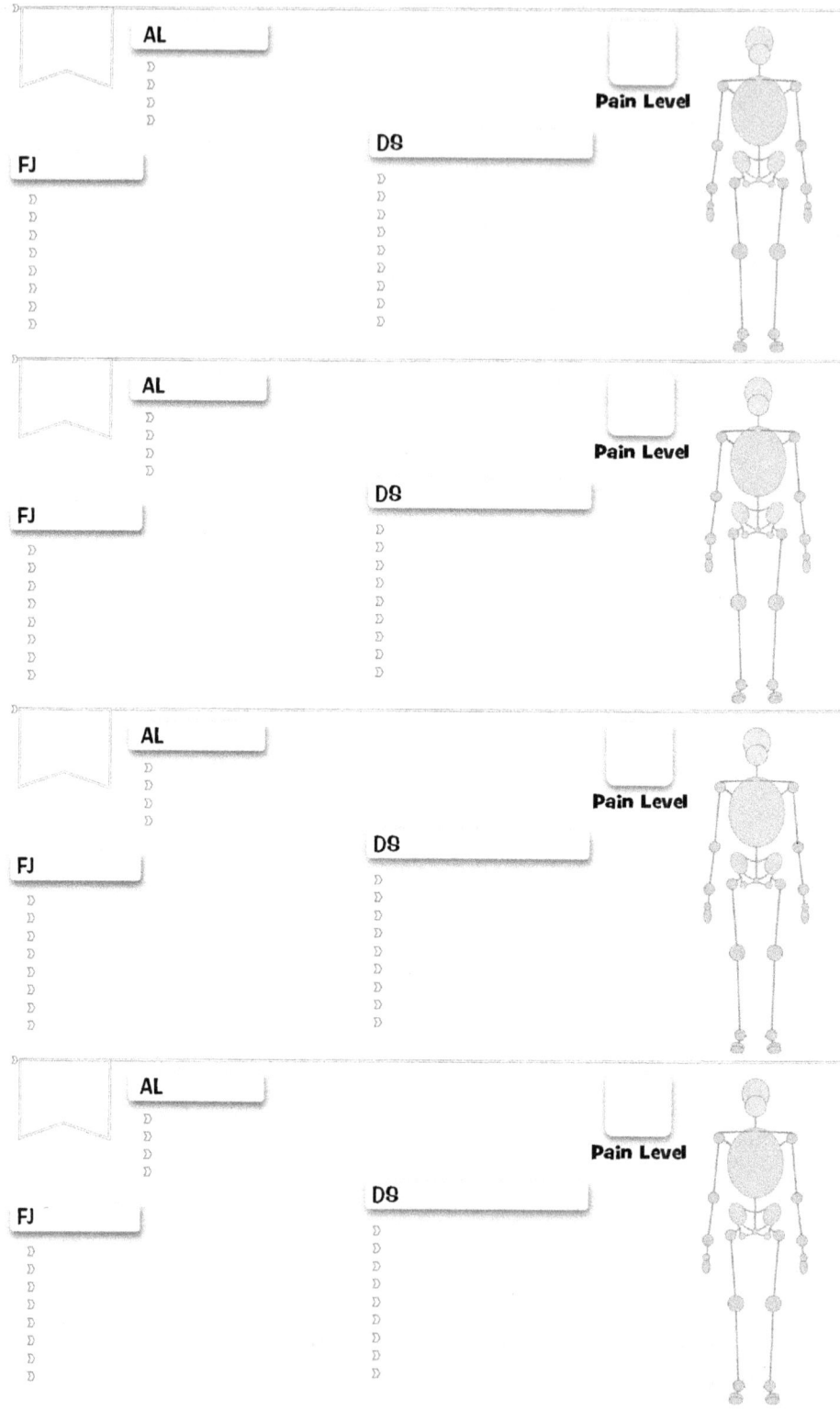

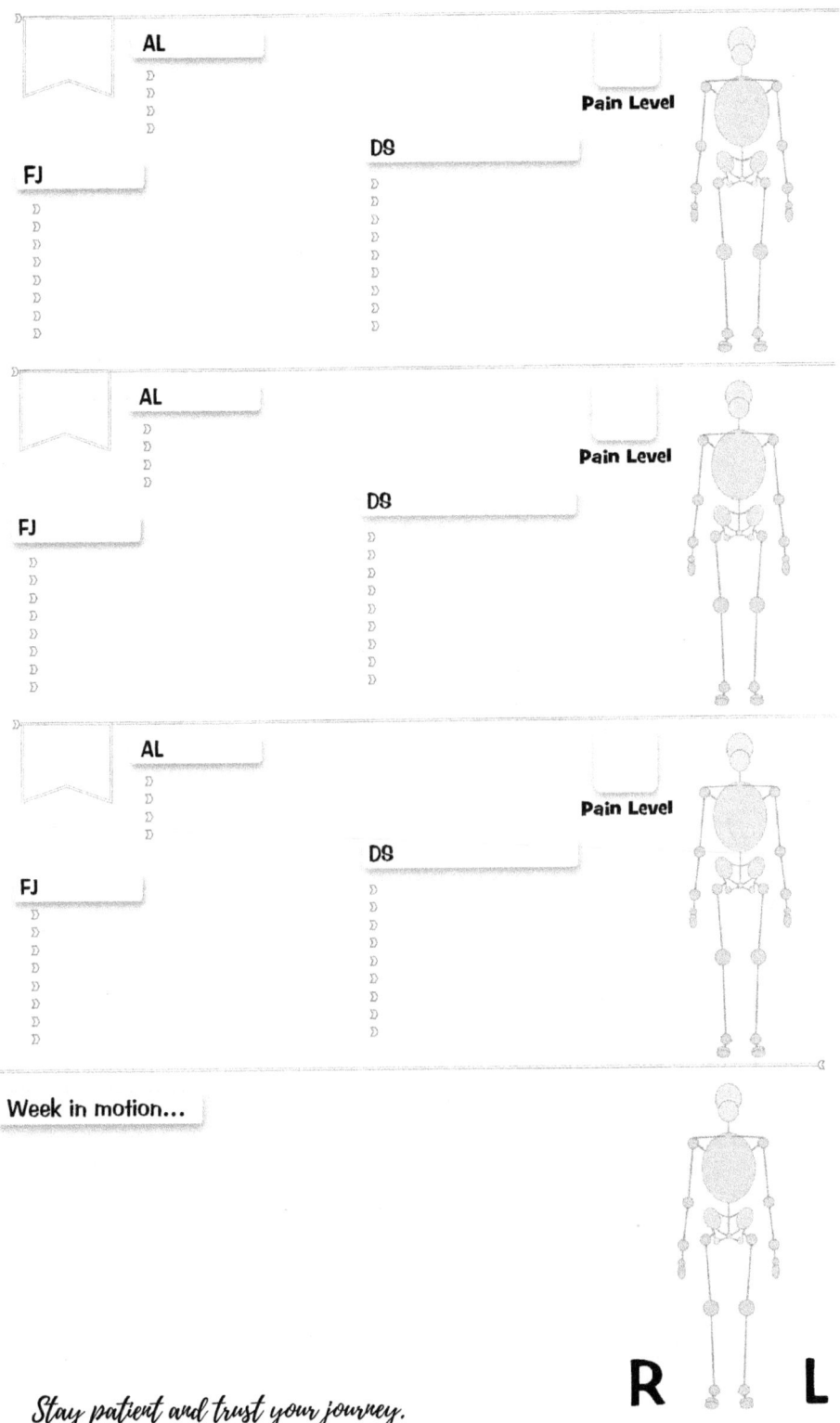

AL

FJ

DS

Pain Level

AL

FJ

DS

Pain Level

AL

FJ

DS

Pain Level

Week in motion...

Stay patient and trust your journey.

R **L**

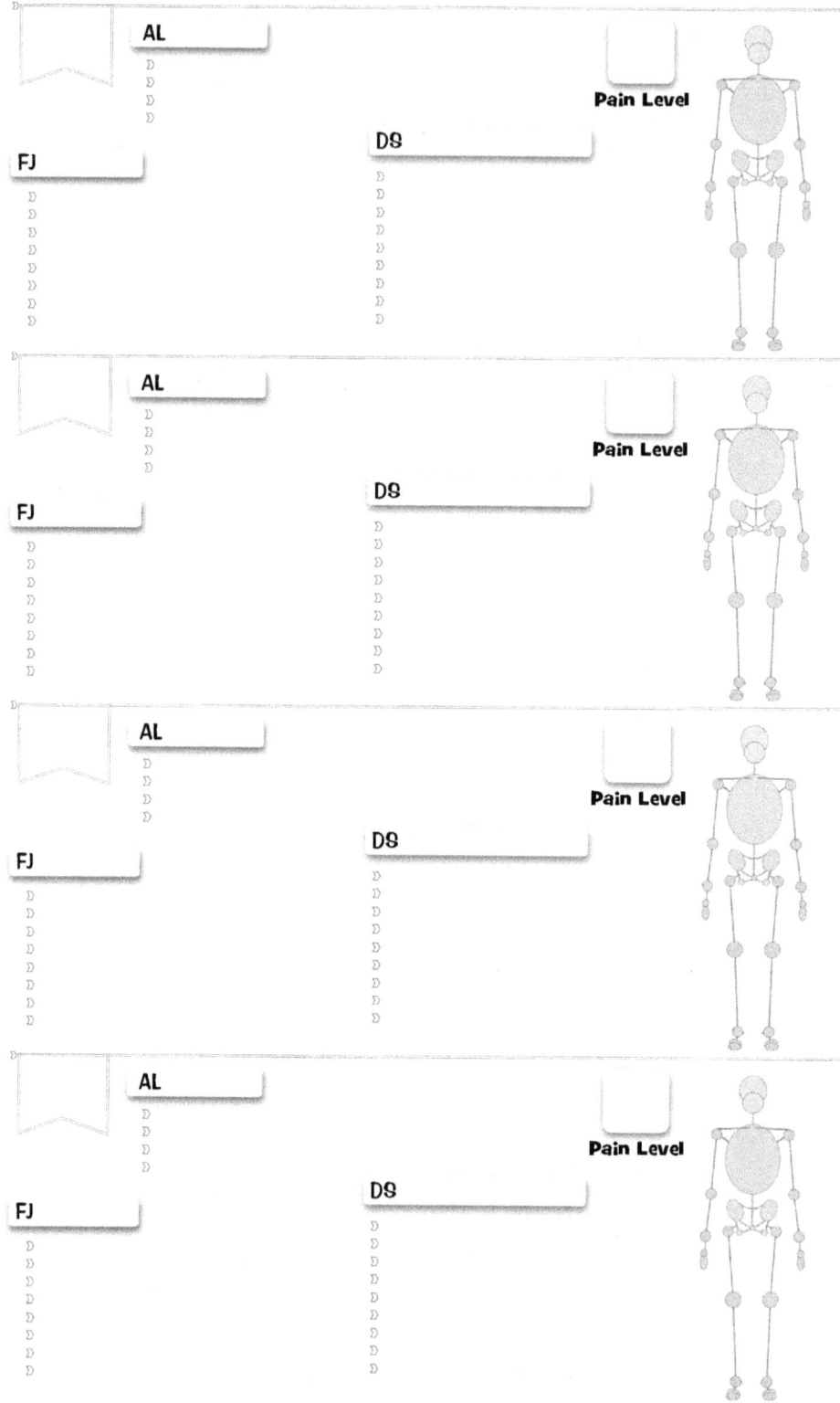

AL

FJ

DS

Pain Level

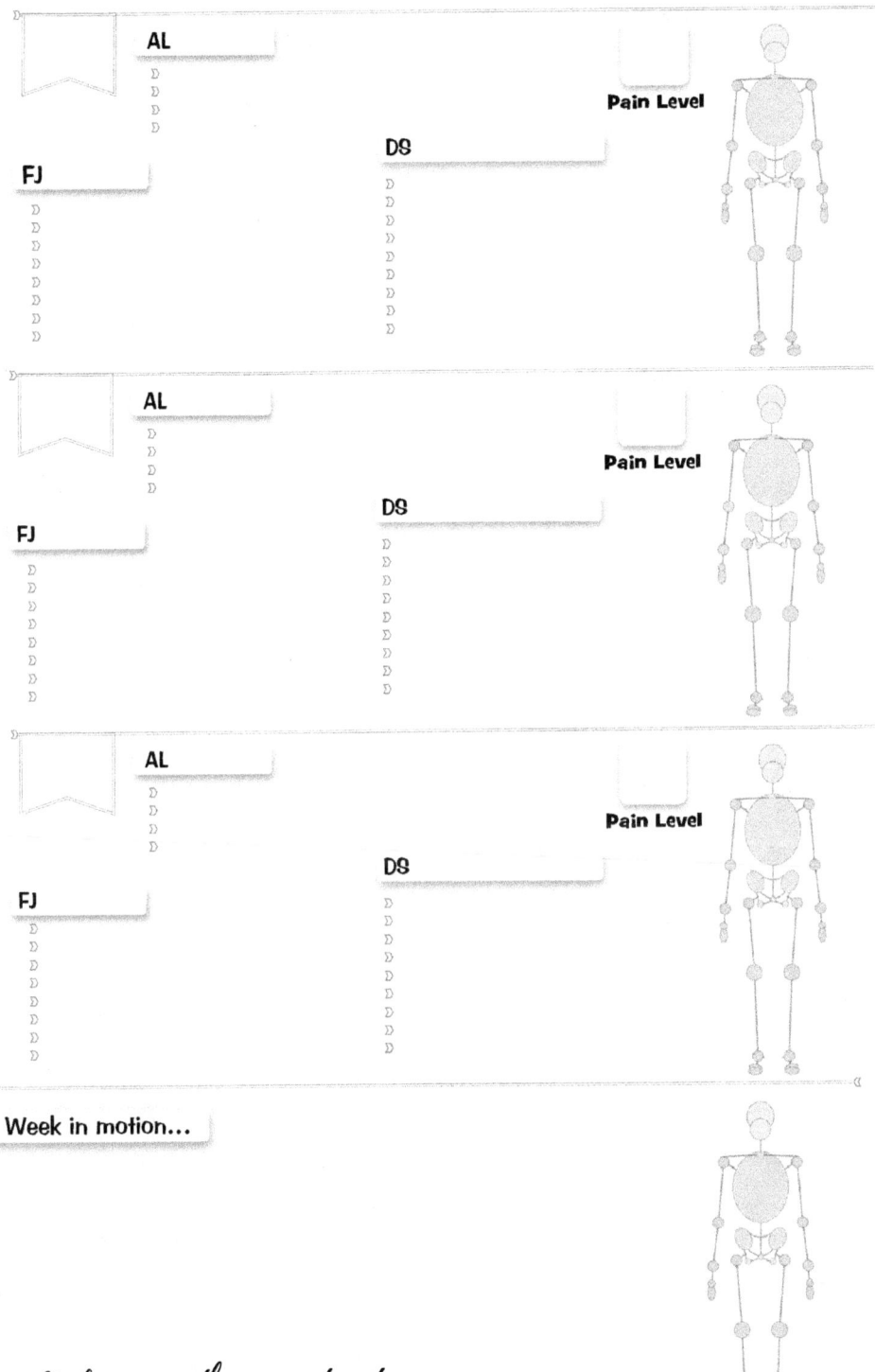

AL
-)
-)
-)
-)

Pain Level

FJ
-)
-)
-)
-)
-)
-)
-)

DS
-)
-)
-)
-)
-)
-)
-)

AL
-)
-)
-)
-)

Pain Level

FJ
-)
-)
-)
-)
-)
-)
-)

DS
-)
-)
-)
-)
-)
-)
-)

AL
-)
-)
-)
-)

Pain Level

FJ
-)
-)
-)
-)
-)
-)
-)

DS
-)
-)
-)
-)
-)
-)
-)

Week in motion...

Make peace with your past so it won't disturb your present. – UNK

R   **L**

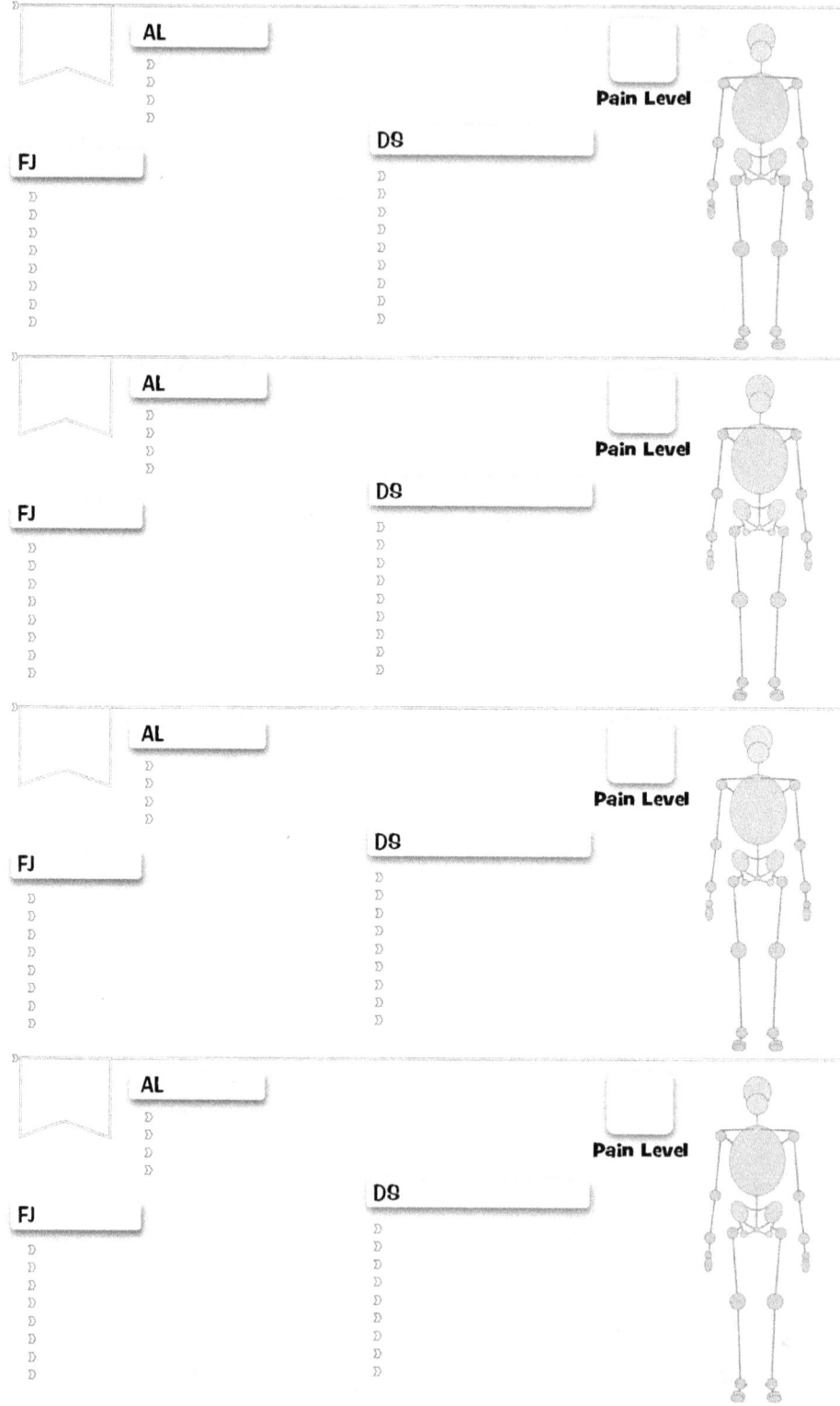

AL

> D
> D
> D
> D

Pain Level

DS

> D
> D
> D
> D
> D
> D
> D

FJ

> D
> D
> D
> D
> D
> D
> D

AL

> D
> D
> D
> D

Pain Level

DS

> D
> D
> D
> D
> D
> D

FJ

> D
> D
> D
> D
> D
> D

AL

> D
> D
> D
> D

Pain Level

DS

> D
> D
> D
> D
> D
> D
> D

FJ

> D
> D
> D
> D
> D
> D
> D

Week in motion...

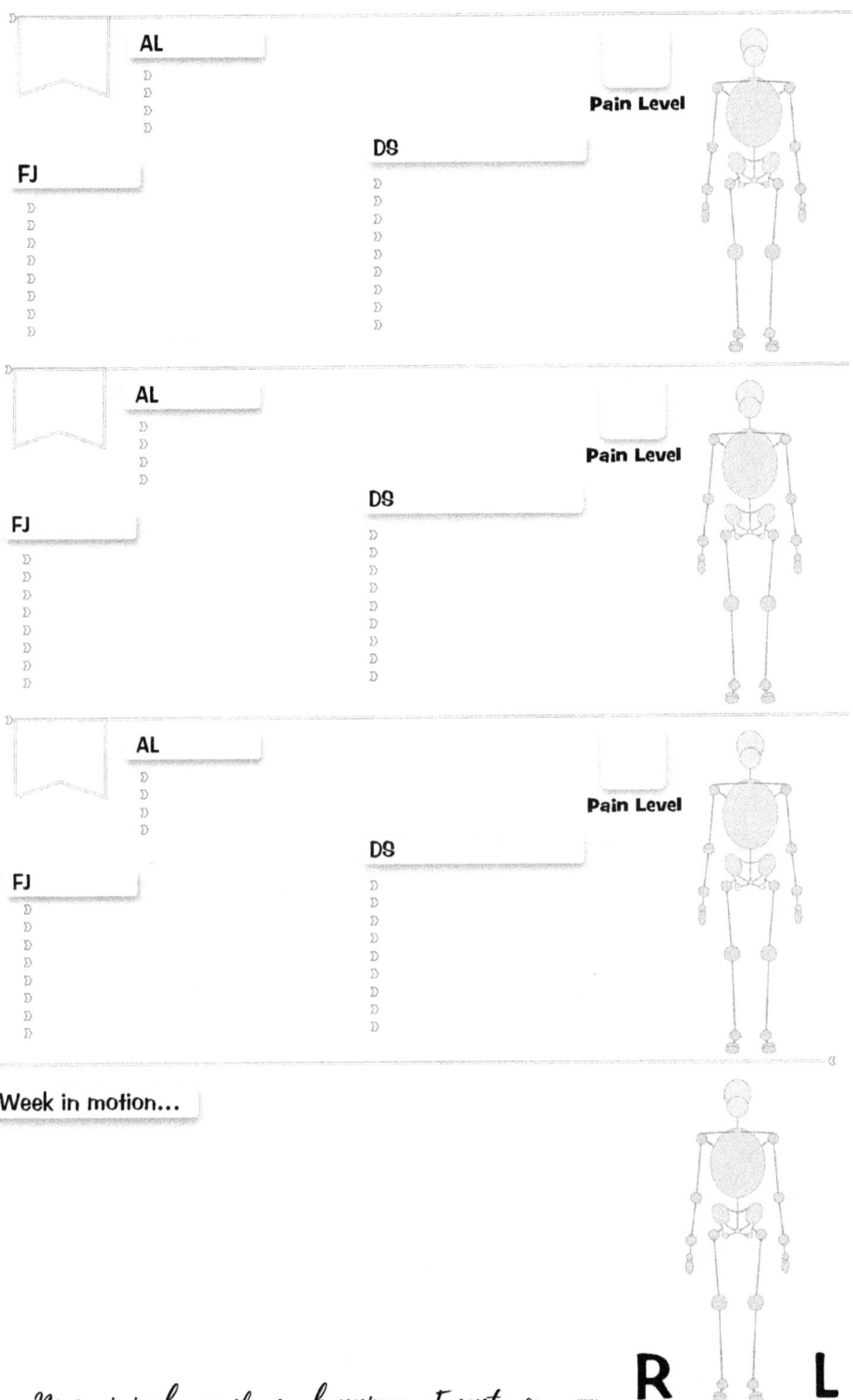

R　　**L**

No one is in charge of your happiness. Except you. – UNK

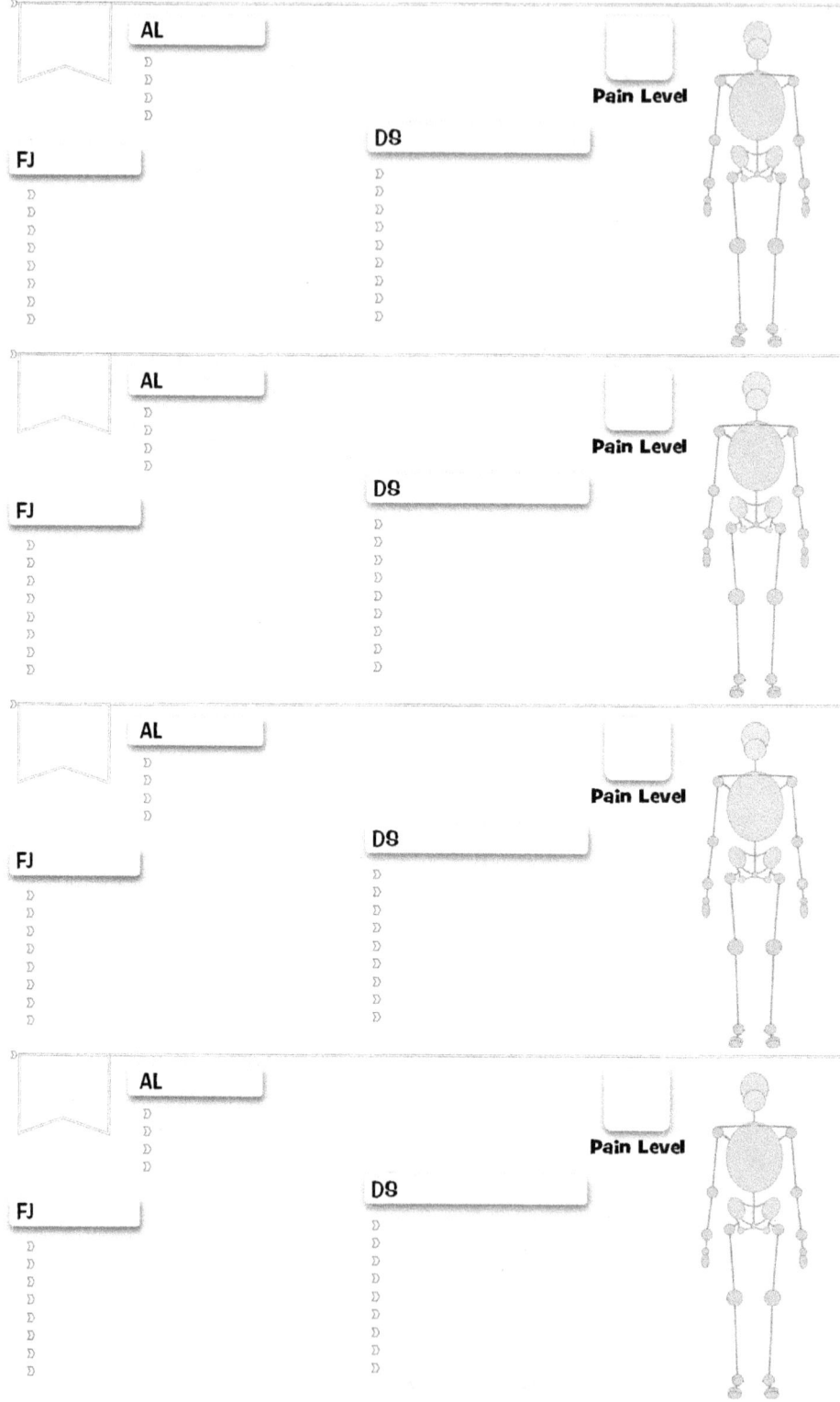

AL

FJ

DS

Pain Level

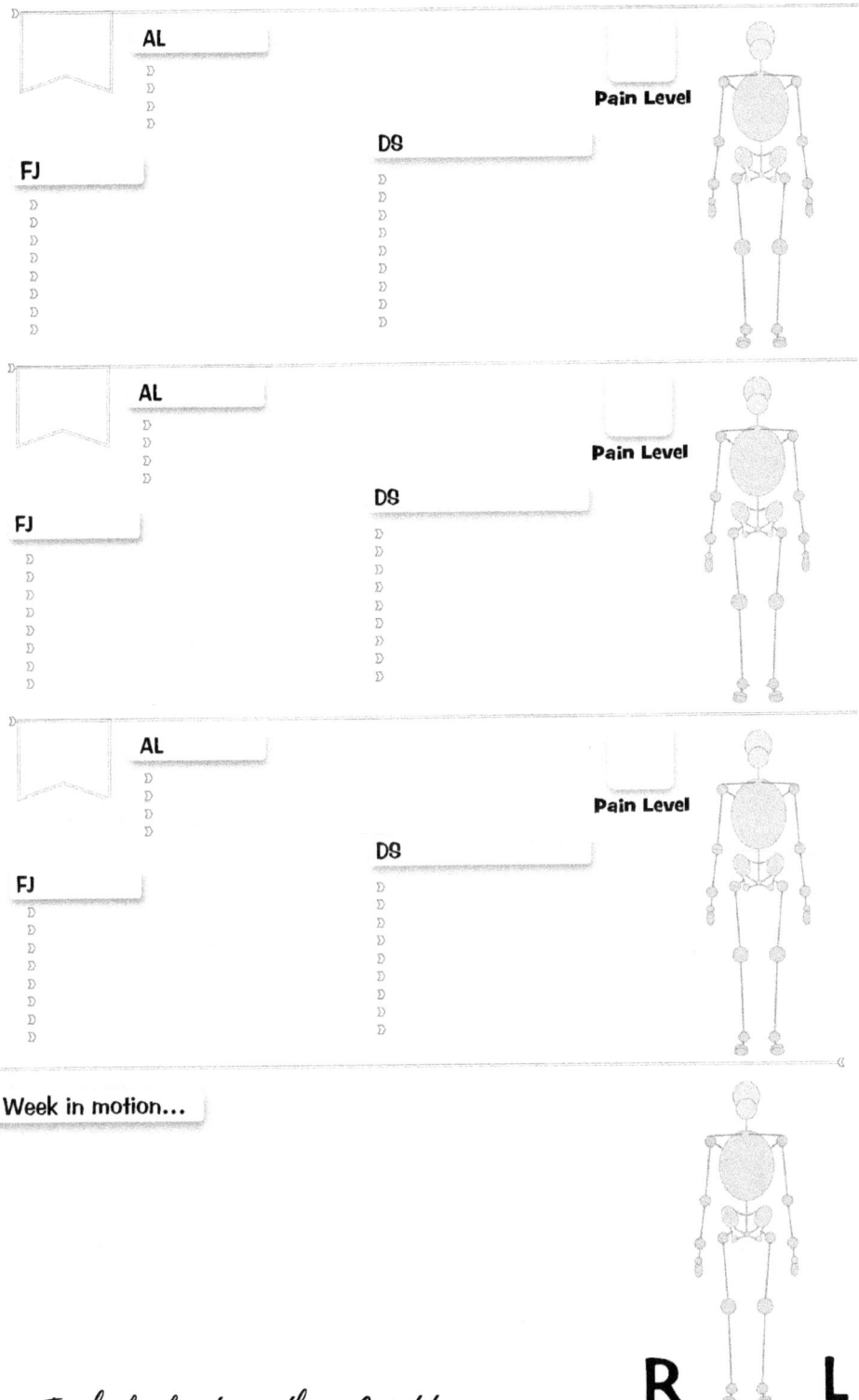

AL

Pain Level

FJ

DS

AL

Pain Level

FJ

DS

AL

Pain Level

FJ

DS

Week in motion...

R   L

Time heals almost everything. Give it time. – UNK

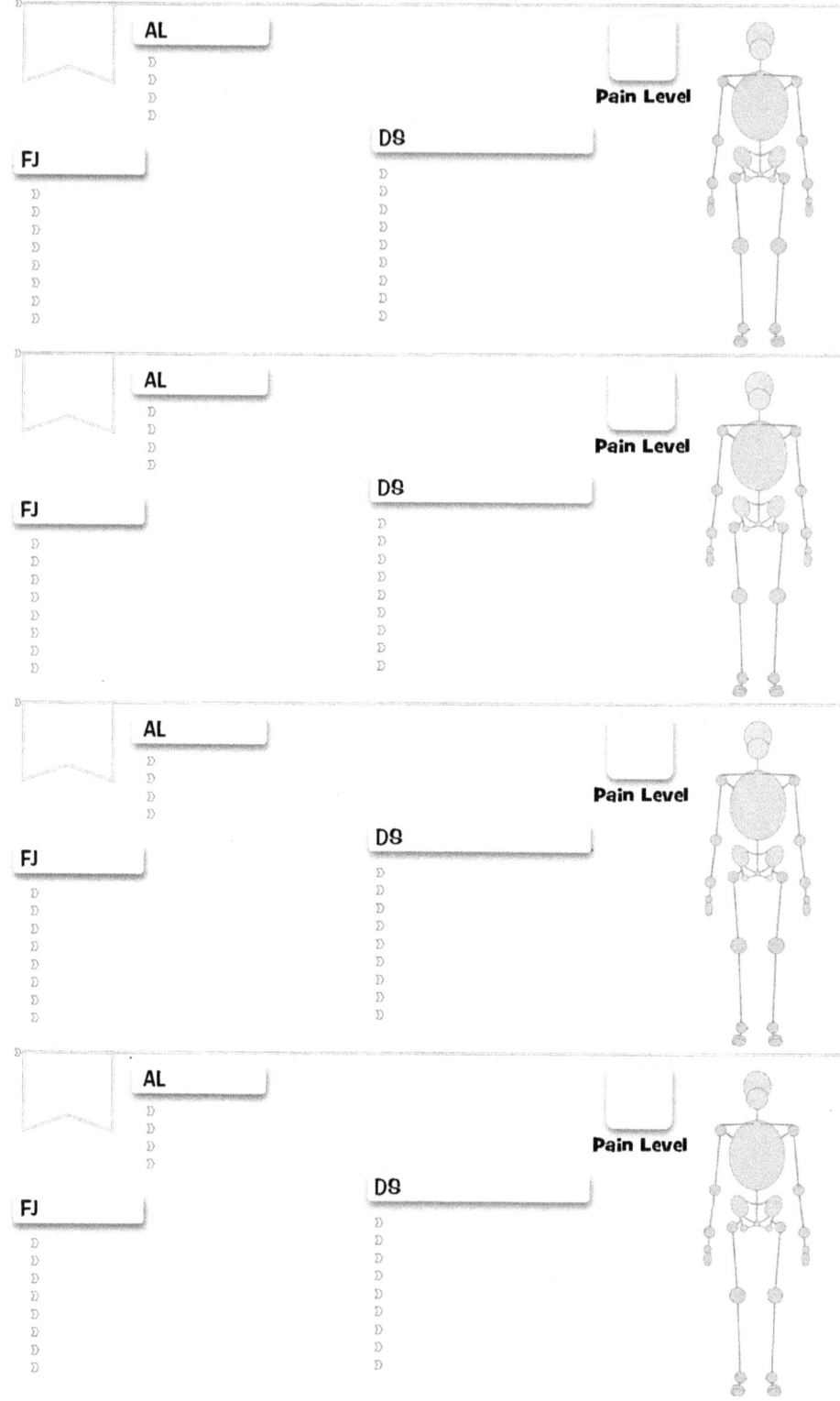

AL

FJ

DS

Pain Level

AL

FJ

DS

Pain Level

AL

FJ

DS

Pain Level

AL

FJ

DS

Pain Level

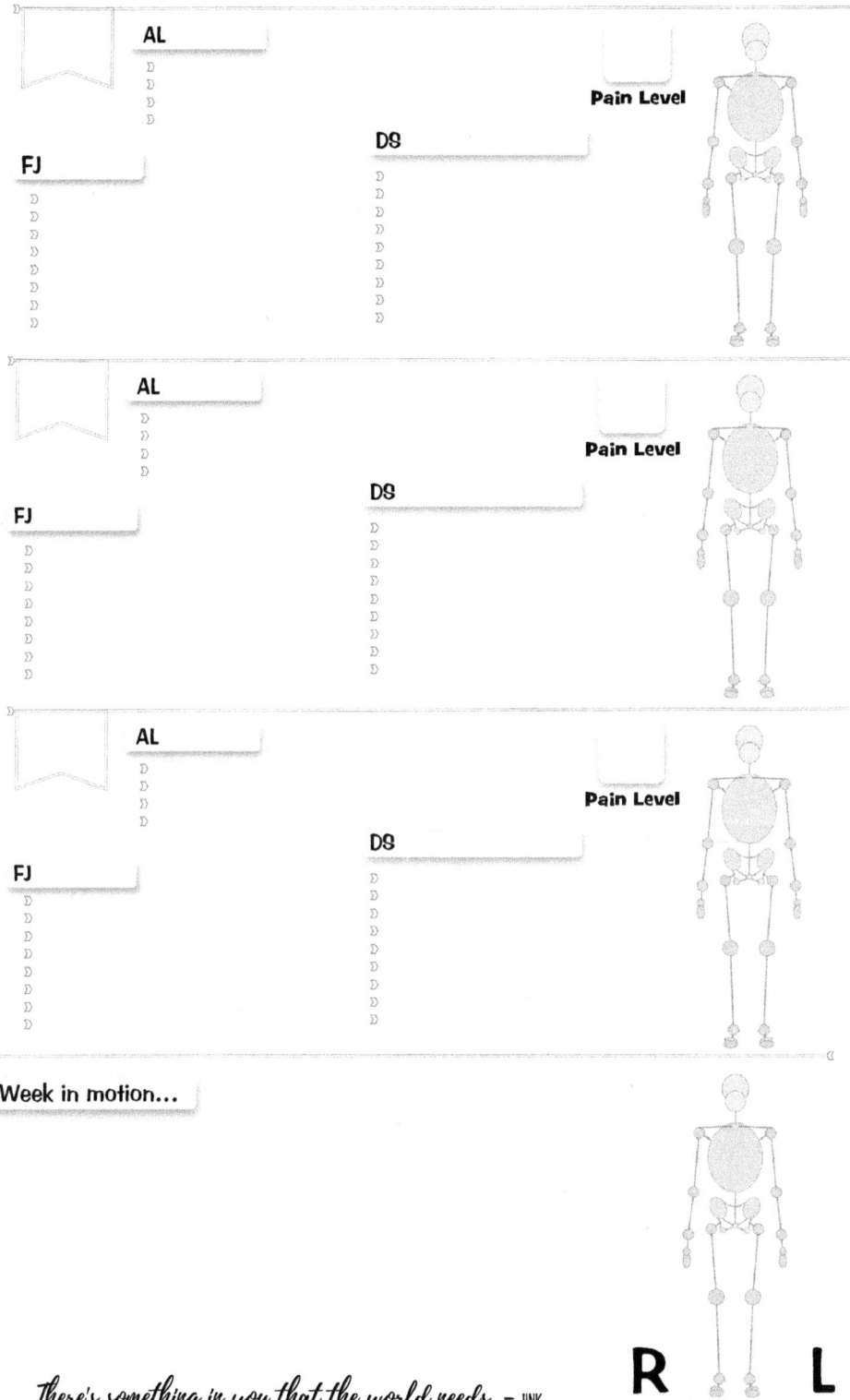

AL
- D
- D
- D
- D

Pain Level

FJ
- D
- D
- D
- D
- D
- D
- D

DS
- D
- D
- D
- D
- D
- D
- D

AL
- D
- D
- D
- D

Pain Level

FJ
- D
- D
- D
- D
- D
- D
- D

DS
- D
- D
- D
- D
- D
- D
- D

AL
- D
- D
- D
- D

Pain Level

FJ
- D
- D
- D
- D
- D
- D
- D

DS
- D
- D
- D
- D
- D
- D
- D

Week in motion...

R   L

There's something in you that the world needs. – UNK

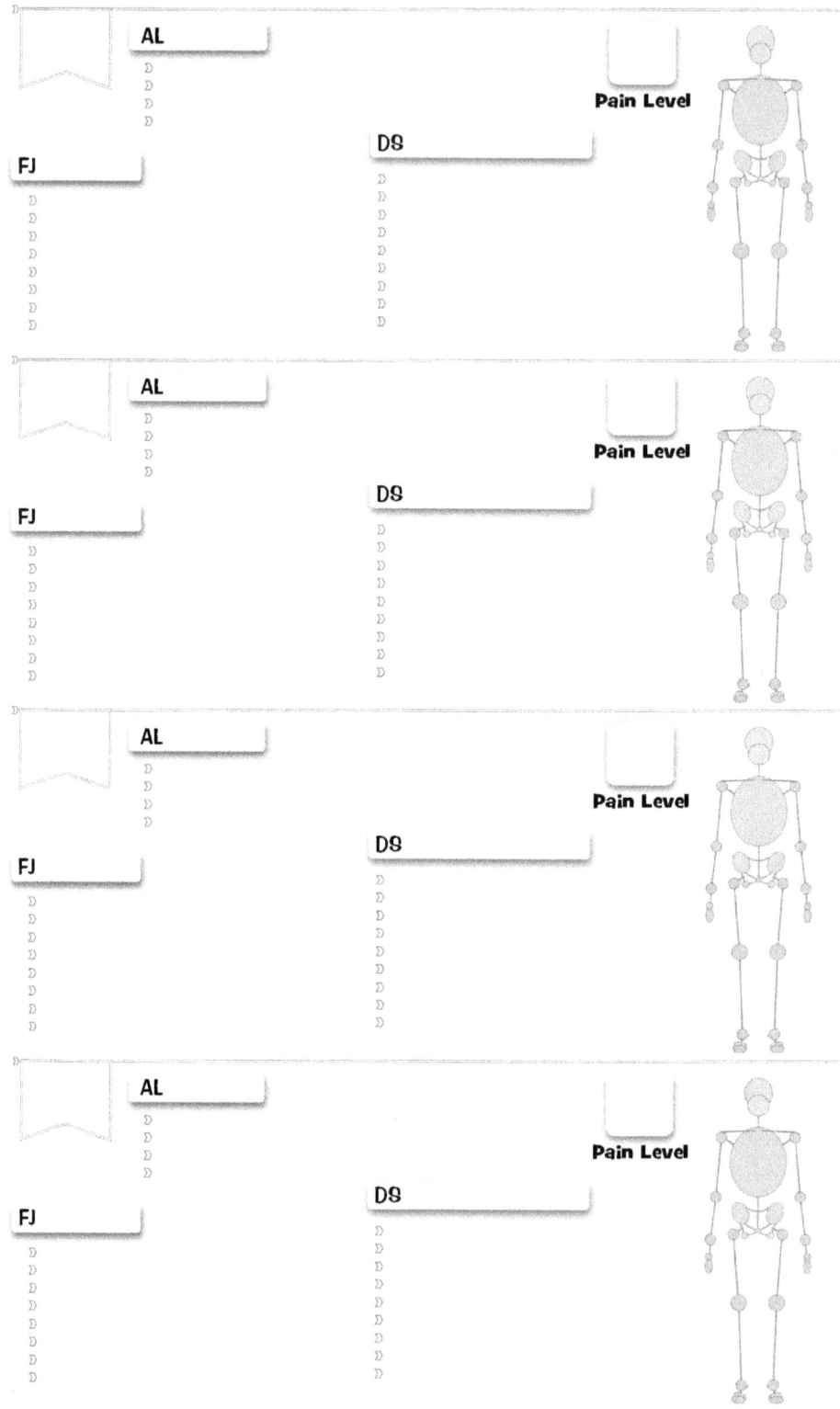

AL

FJ

DS

Pain Level

AL

FJ

DS

Pain Level

AL

FJ

DS

Pain Level

AL

FJ

DS

Pain Level

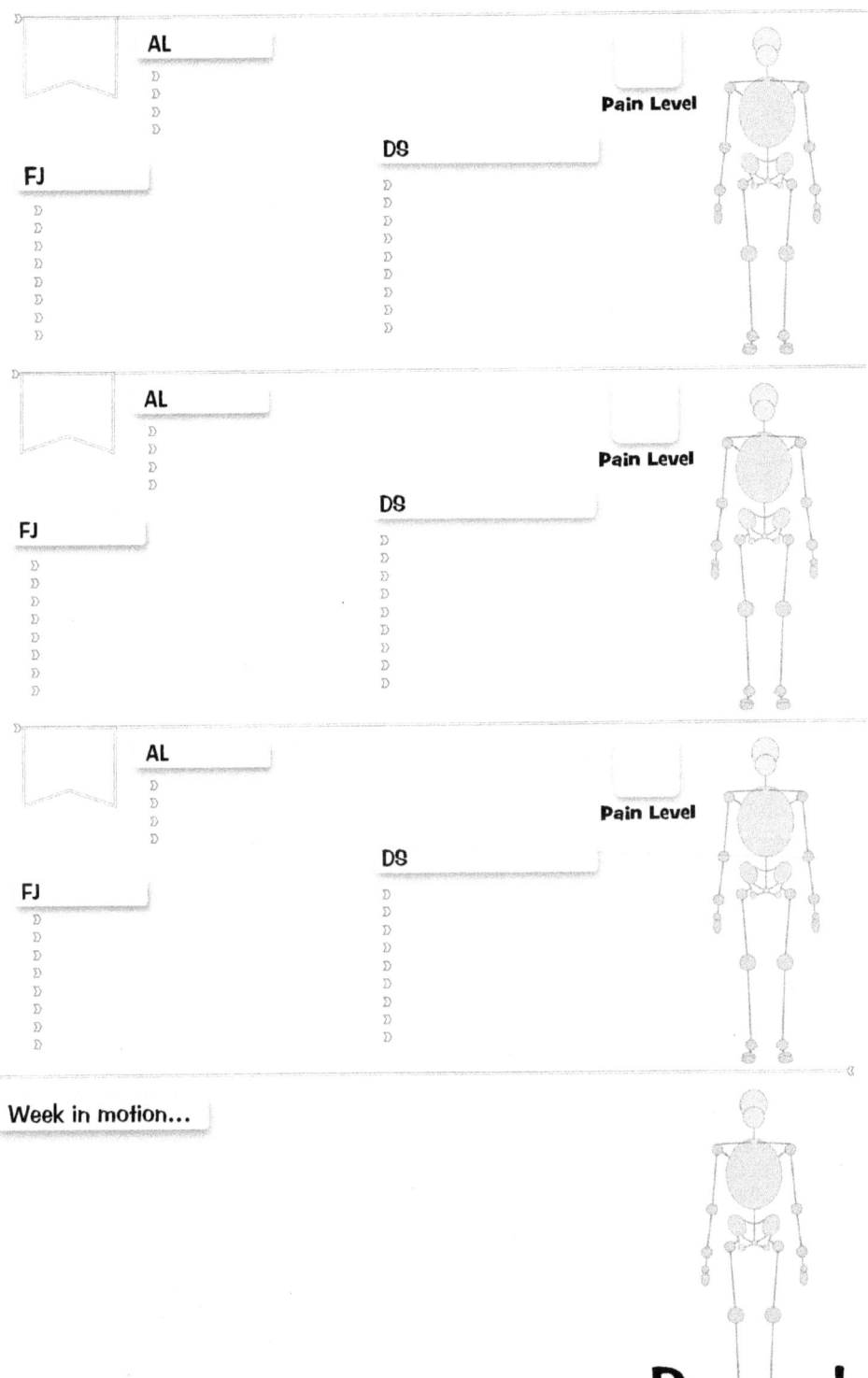

AL

FJ

DS

Pain Level

AL

FJ

DS

Pain Level

AL

FJ

DS

Pain Level

Week in motion...

A grateful heart is a magnet for miracles. —UNK

R **L**

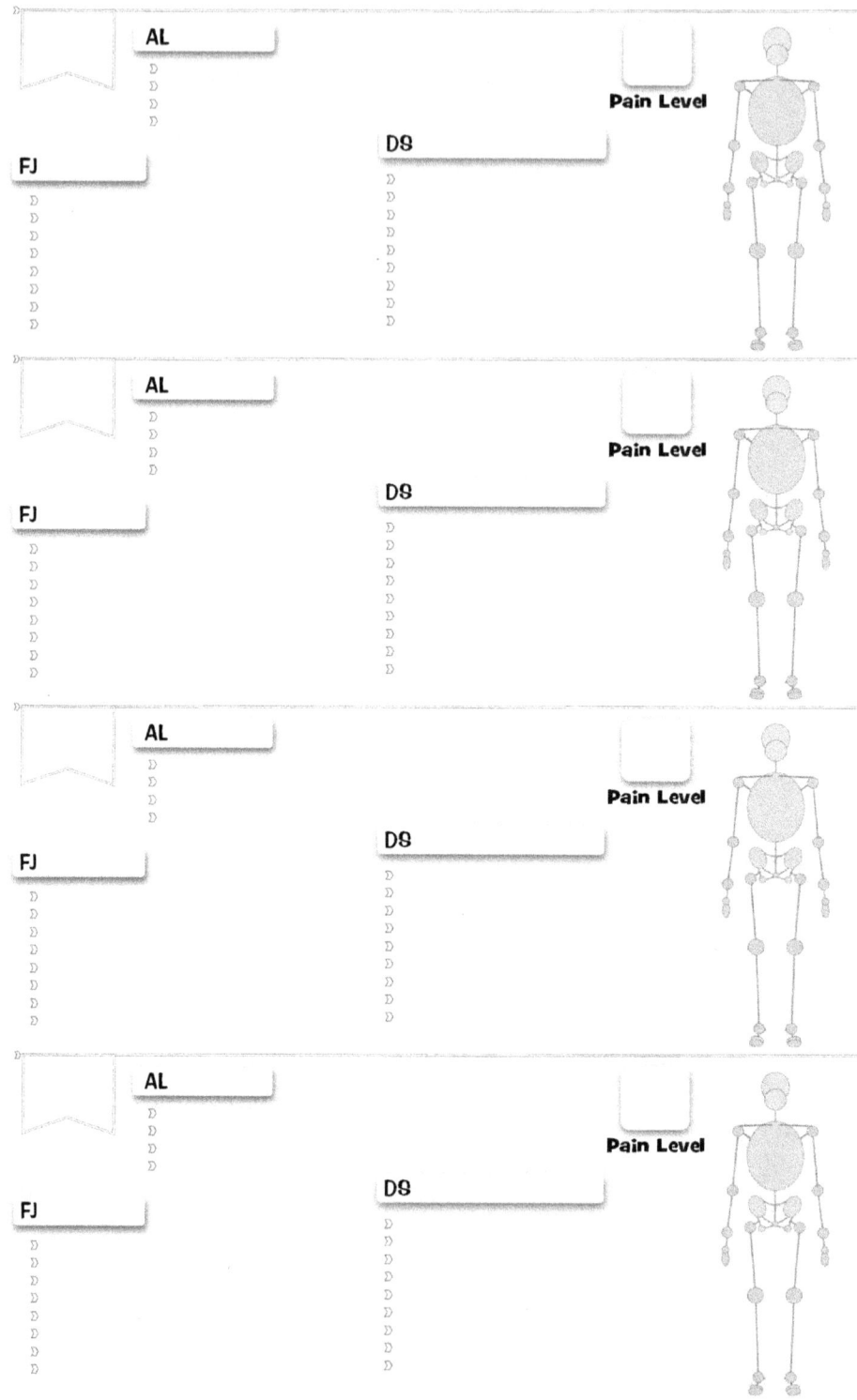

AL

FJ

Pain Level

DS

AL

FJ

Pain Level

DS

AL

FJ

Pain Level

DS

AL

FJ

Pain Level

DS

AL
-)
-)
-)
-)

Pain Level

FJ
-)
-)
-)
-)
-)
-)
-)

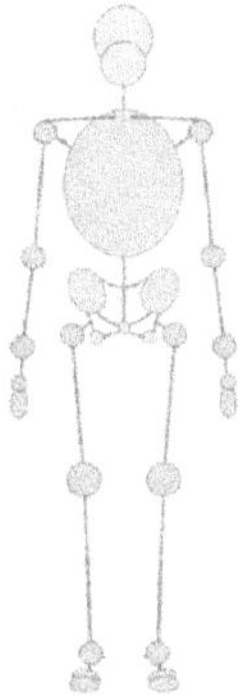

DS
-)
-)
-)
-)
-)
-)
-)

AL
-)
-)
-)
-)

Pain Level

FJ
-)
-)
-)
-)
-)
-)

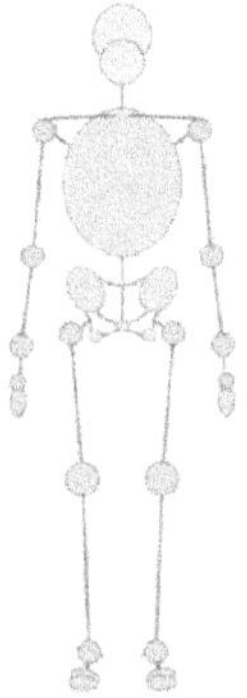

DS
-)
-)
-)
-)
-)
-)

AL
-)
-)
-)
-)

Pain Level

FJ
-)
-)
-)
-)
-)
-)
-)

DS
-)
-)
-)
-)
-)
-)
-)

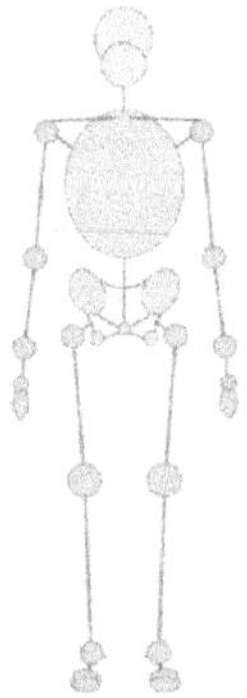

Week in motion...

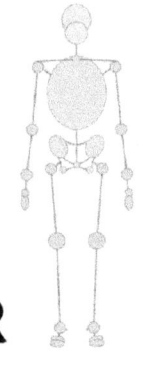

You never need an excuse, or an apology, for why you are taking care of yourself.

R **L**

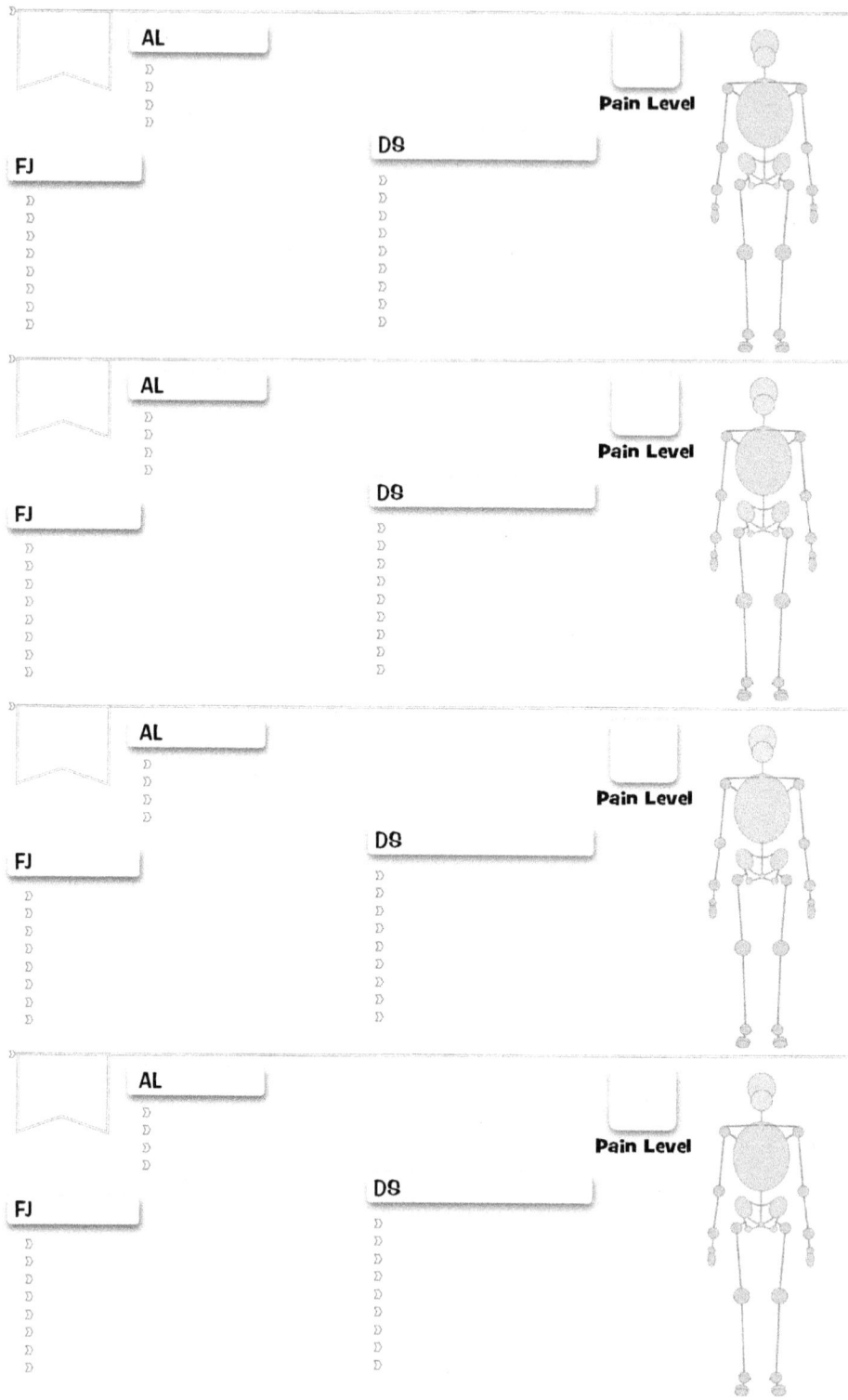

AL
〉
〉
〉
〉

Pain Level

DS
〉
〉
〉
〉
〉
〉
〉

FJ
〉
〉
〉
〉
〉
〉
〉

AL
〉
〉
〉

Pain Level

DS
〉
〉
〉
〉
〉
〉
〉

FJ
〉
〉
〉
〉
〉
〉
〉

AL
〉
〉
〉

Pain Level

DS
〉
〉
〉
〉
〉
〉
〉

FJ
〉
〉
〉
〉
〉
〉
〉

AL
〉
〉
〉
〉

Pain Level

DS
〉
〉
〉
〉
〉
〉
〉

FJ
〉
〉
〉
〉
〉
〉
〉

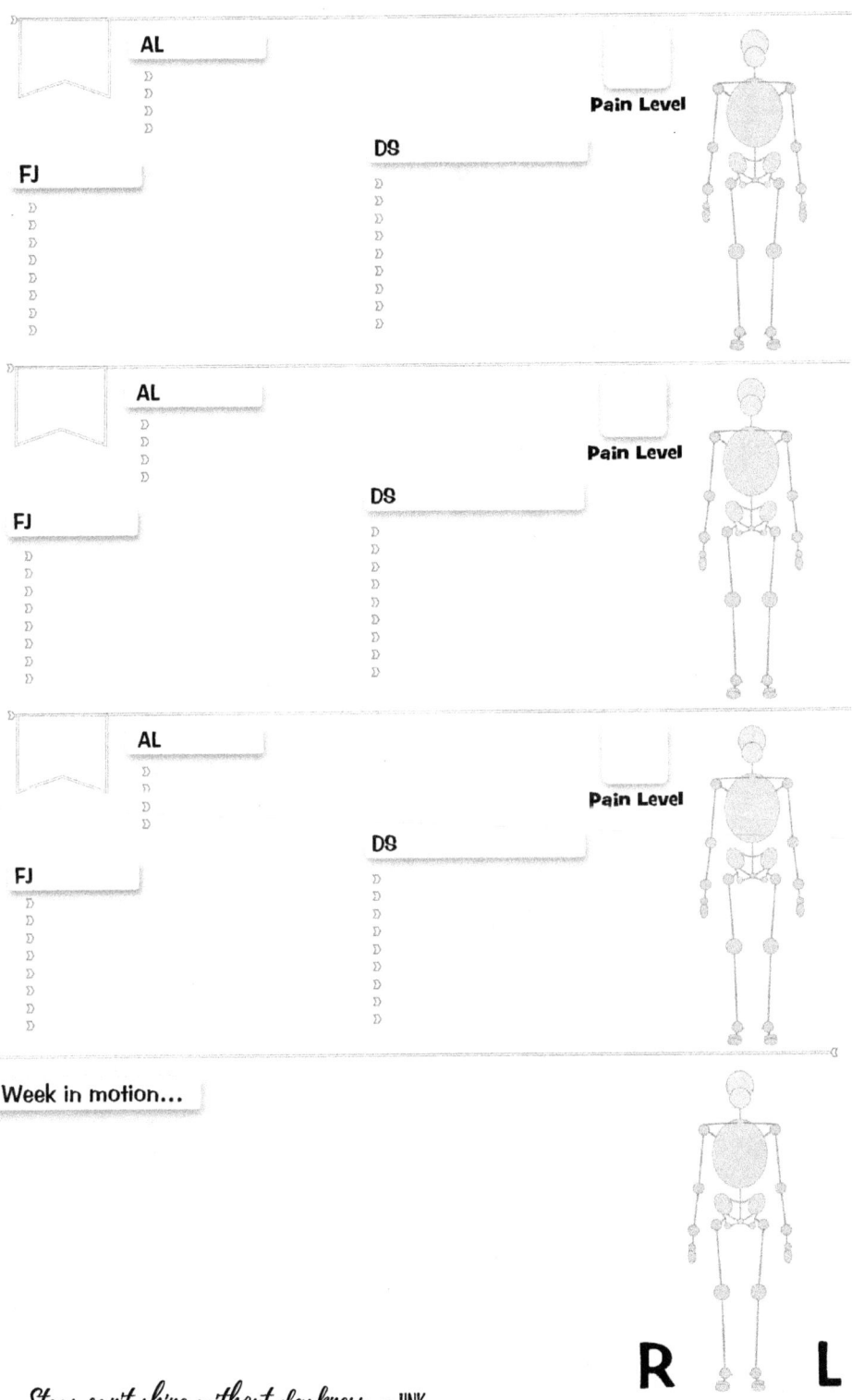

AL

FJ

DS

Pain Level

AL

FJ

DS

Pain Level

AL

FJ

DS

Pain Level

Week in motion...

R L

Stars can't shine without darkness. – UNK

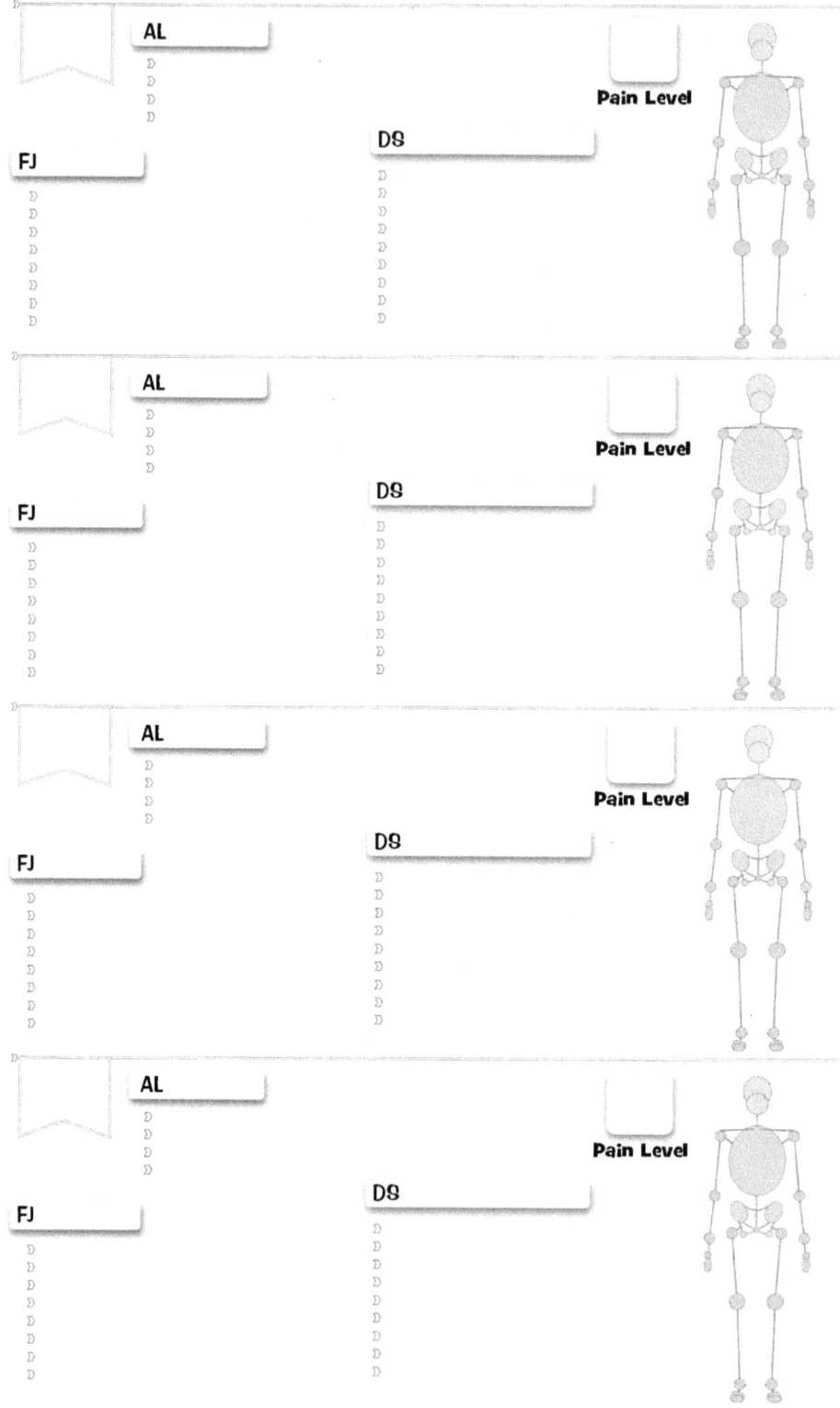

AL

FJ

DS

Pain Level

AL

)
)
)
)

FJ

)
)
)
)
)
)
)

DS

)
)
)
)
)
)
)
)

Pain Level

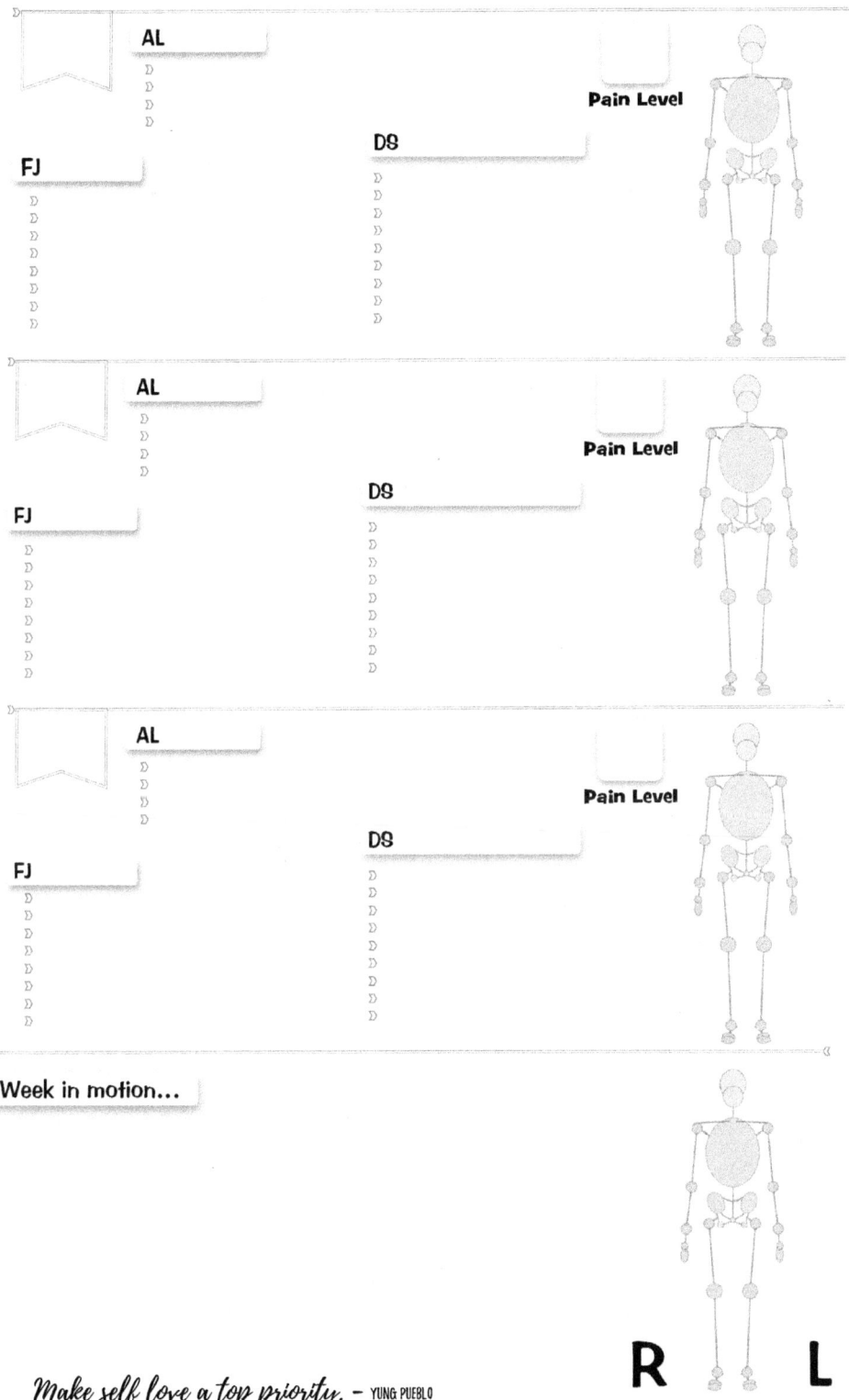

AL

)
)
)
)

FJ

)
)
)
)
)
)
)

DS

)
)
)
)
)
)
)

Pain Level

AL

)
)
)
)

FJ

)
)
)
)
)
)
)

DS

)
)
)
)
)
)
)

Pain Level

Week in motion...

R   L

Make self love a top priority. — YUNG PUEBLO

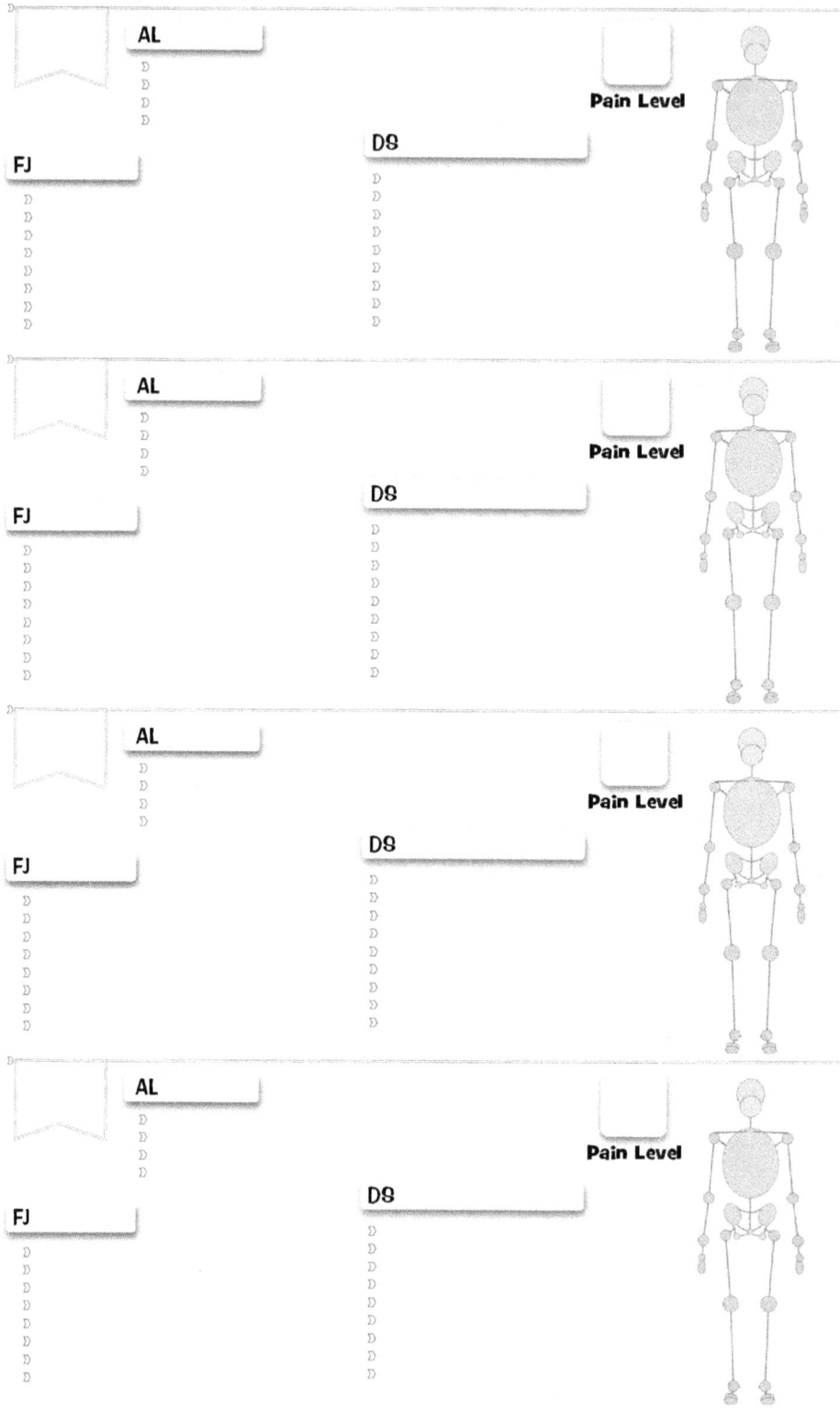

AL

FJ

DS

Pain Level

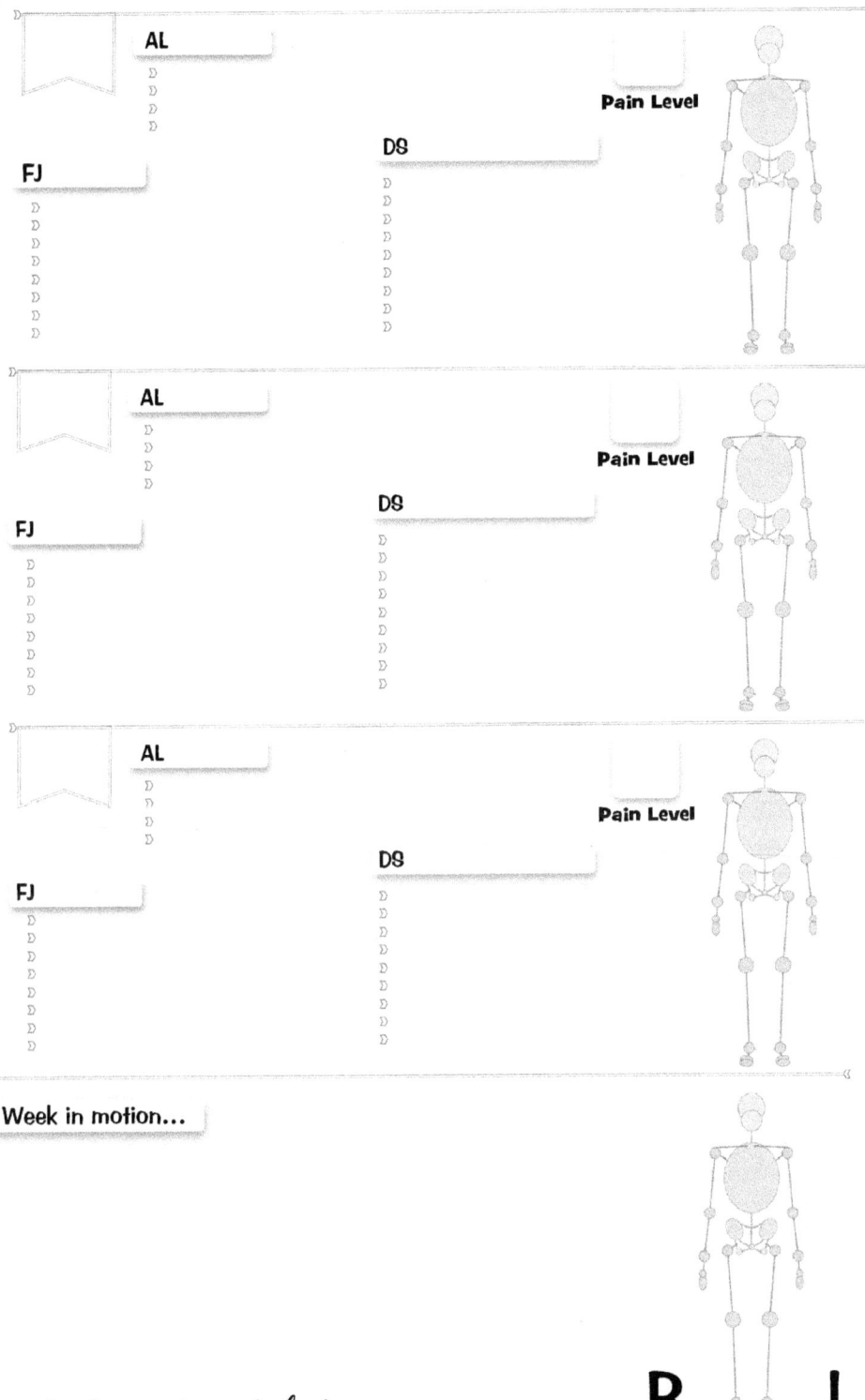

AL

Pain Level

DS

FJ

AL

Pain Level

DS

FJ

AL

Pain Level

DS

FJ

Week in motion...

Create space for daily healing. – YUNG PUEBLO

R   L

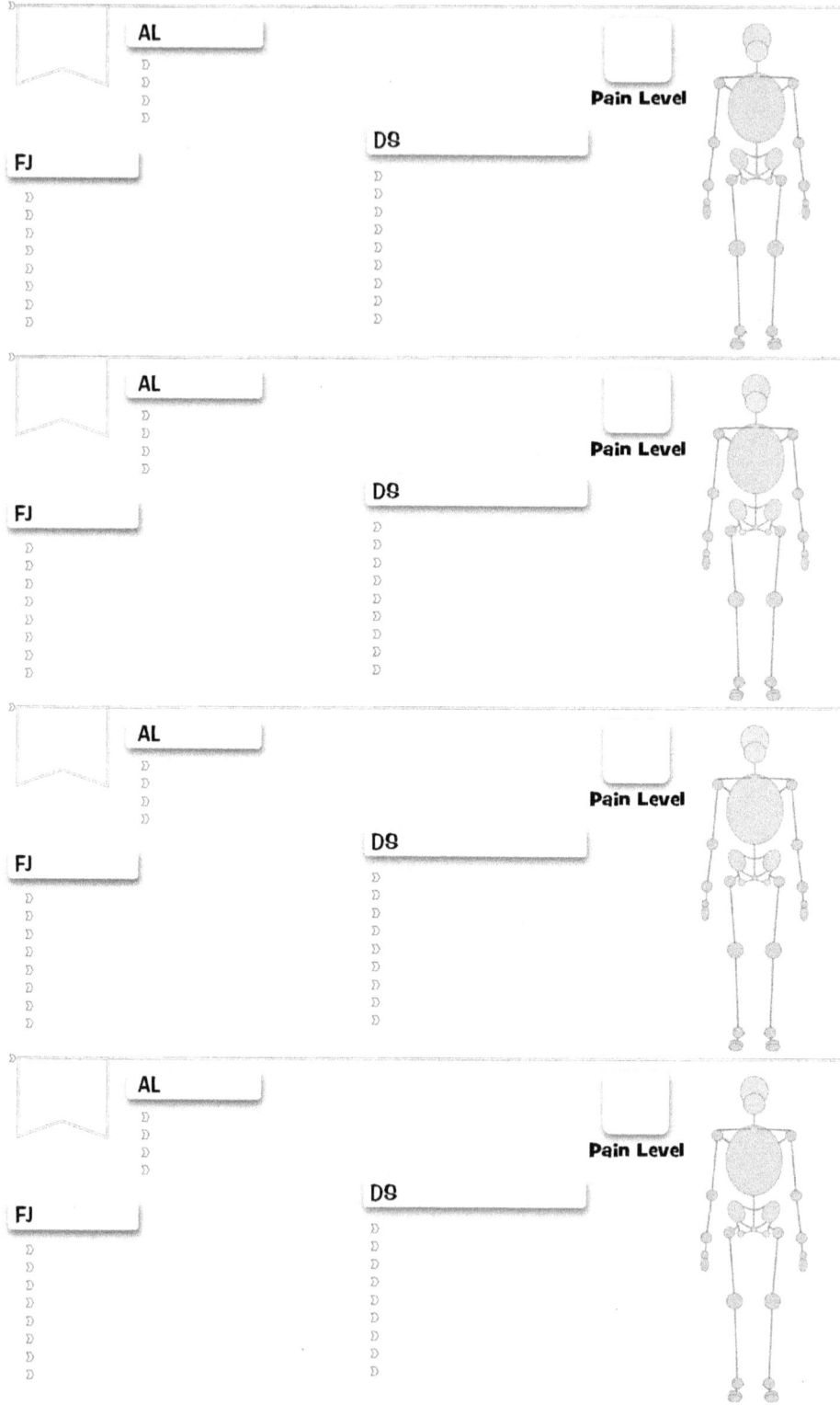

AL

>
>
>
>

FJ

>
>
>
>
>
>
>

DS

>
>
>
>
>
>
>
>

Pain Level

AL

>
>
>
>

FJ

>
>
>
>
>
>
>

DS

>
>
>
>
>
>

Pain Level

AL

>
>
>
>

FJ

>
>
>
>
>
>
>

DS

>
>
>
>
>
>
>

Pain Level

AL

>
>
>
>

FJ

>
>
>
>
>
>
>

DS

>
>
>
>
>
>
>

Pain Level

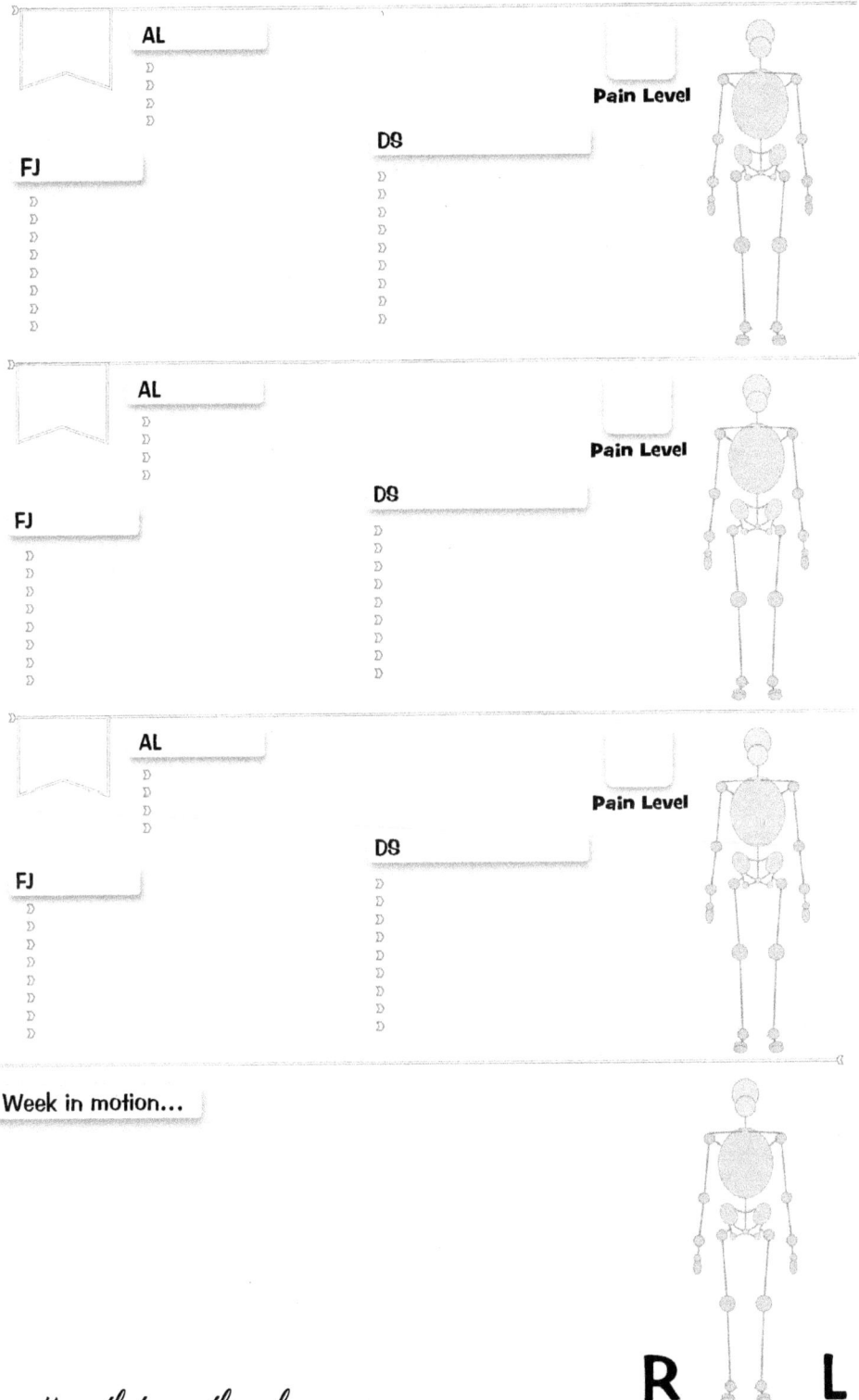

AL

FJ

DS

Pain Level

AL

FJ

DS

Pain Level

AL

FJ

DS

Pain Level

Week in motion...

R   L

Know that everything changes. - YUNG PUEBLO

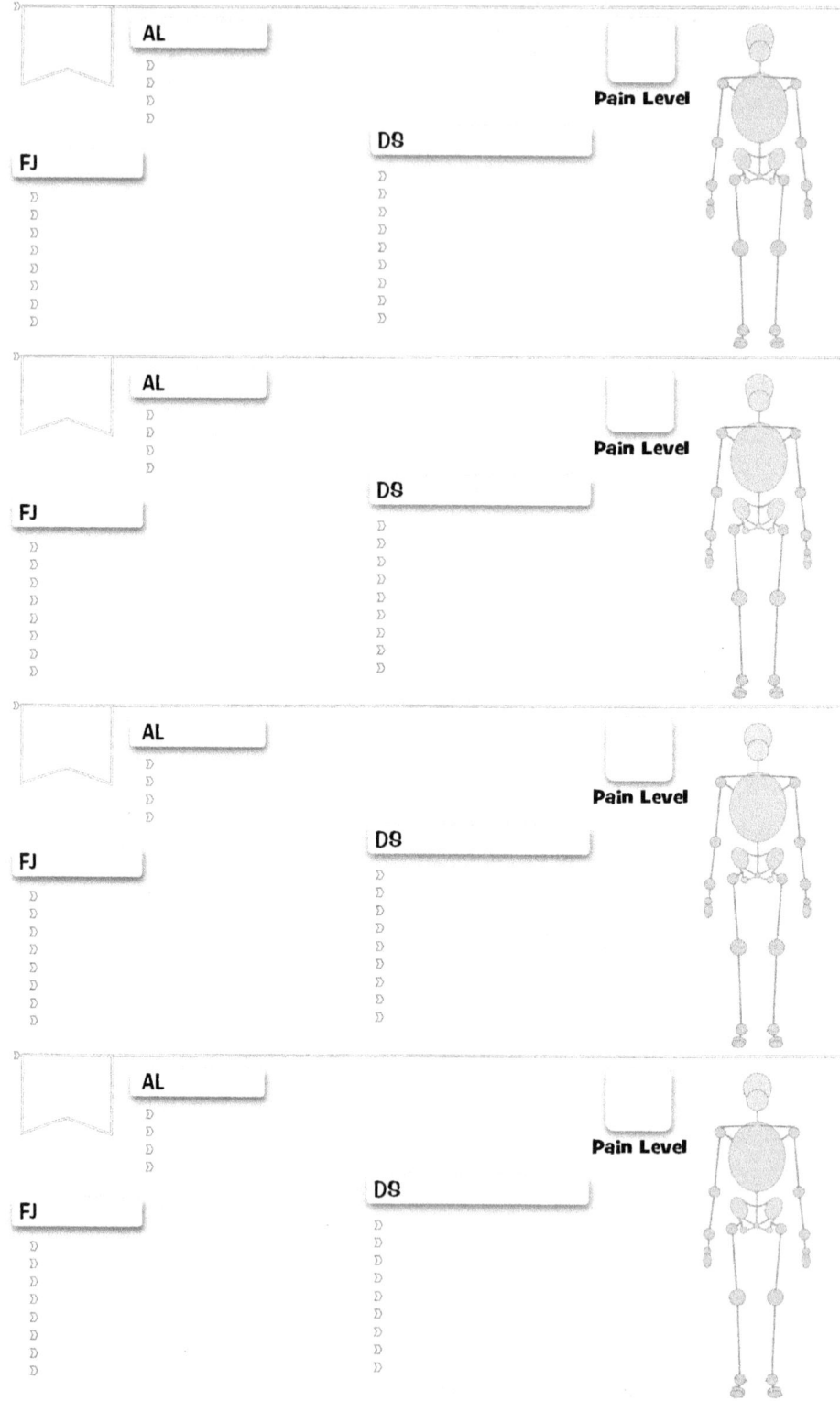

AL

FJ

DS

Pain Level

AL

FJ

DS

Pain Level

AL

FJ

DS

Pain Level

AL

FJ

DS

Pain Level

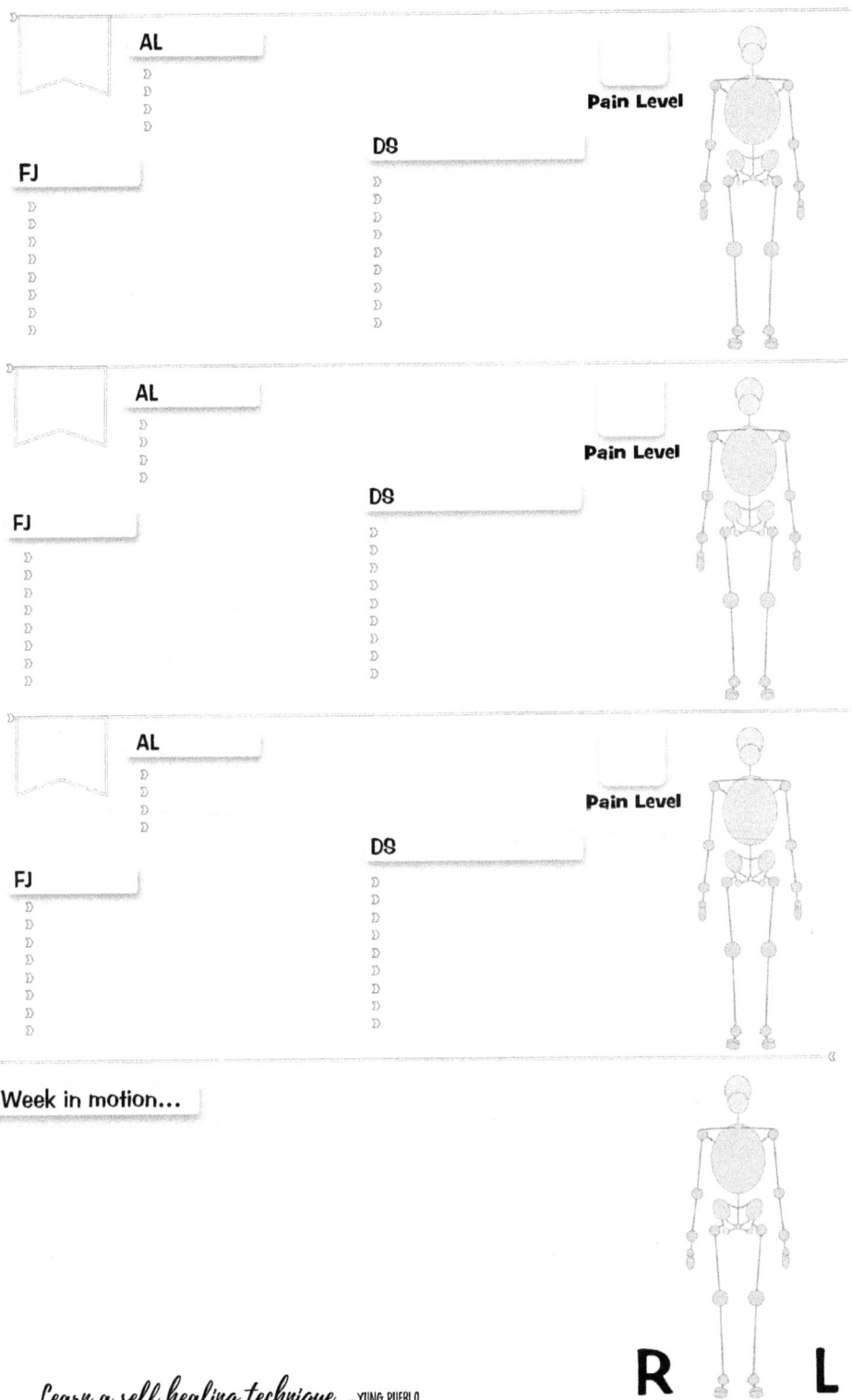

AL

Pain Level

FJ

DS

AL

Pain Level

FJ

DS

AL

Pain Level

FJ

DS

Week in motion...

Learn a self healing technique. - YUNG PUEBLO

R   L

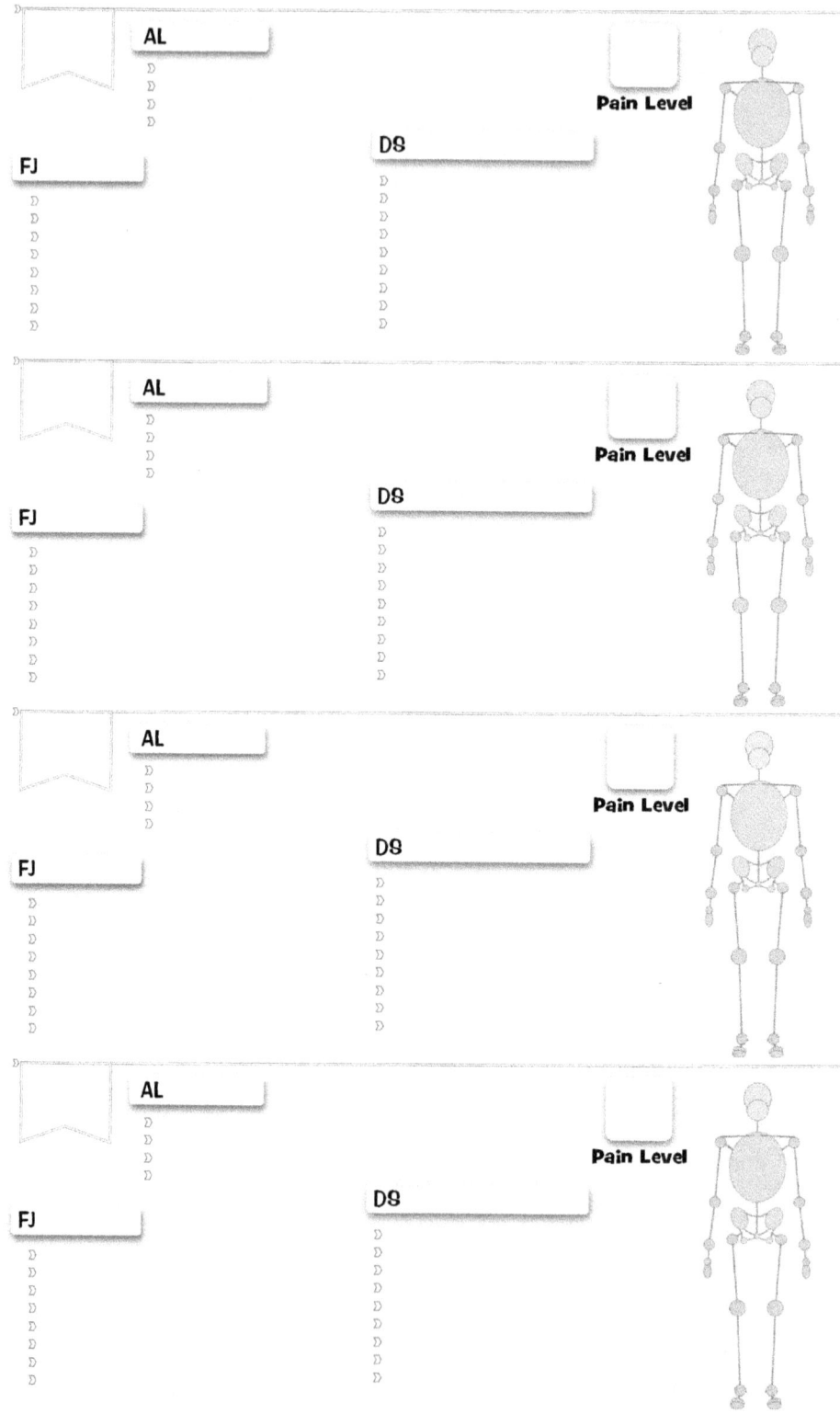

AL

FJ

DS

Pain Level

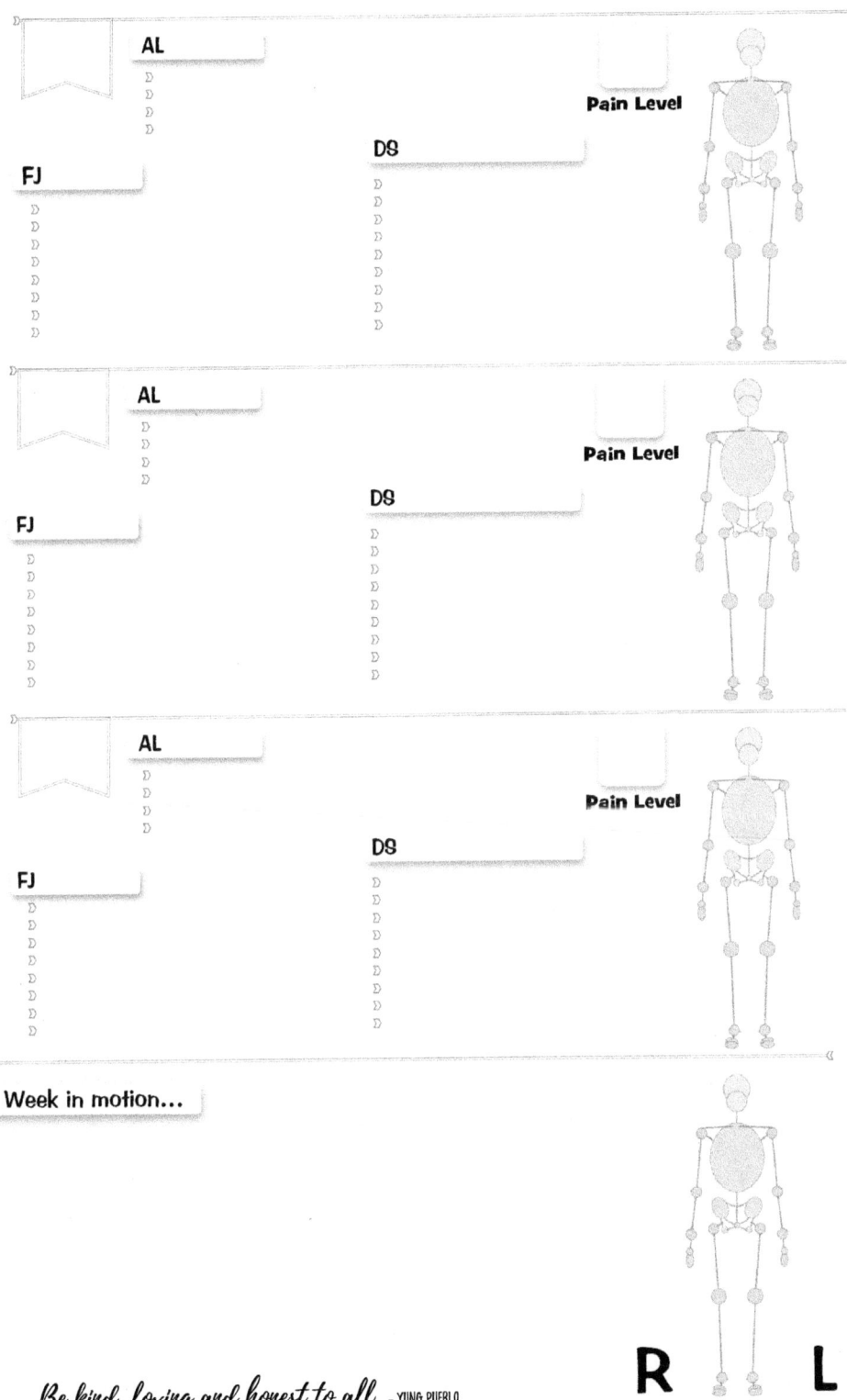

AL
-
-
-
-

FJ
-
-
-
-
-
-
-

DS
-
-
-
-
-
-
-

Pain Level

AL
-
-
-

FJ
-
-
-
-
-
-

DS
-
-
-
-
-
-
-

Pain Level

AL
-
-
-

FJ
-
-
-
-
-
-

DS
-
-
-
-
-
-
-

Pain Level

Week in motion...

Be kind, loving and honest to all. - YUNG PUEBLO

R   L

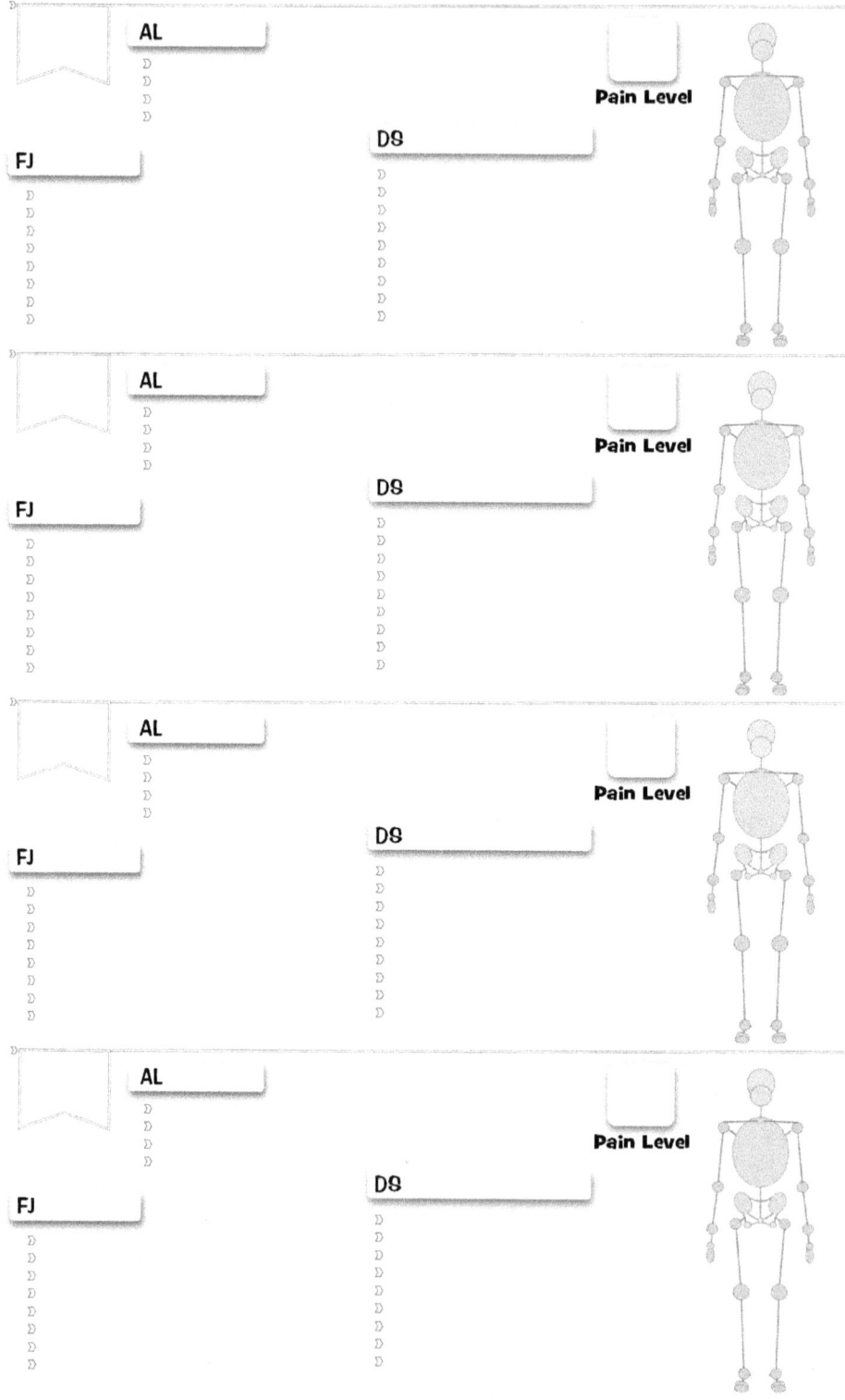

AL

Pain Level

FJ

DS

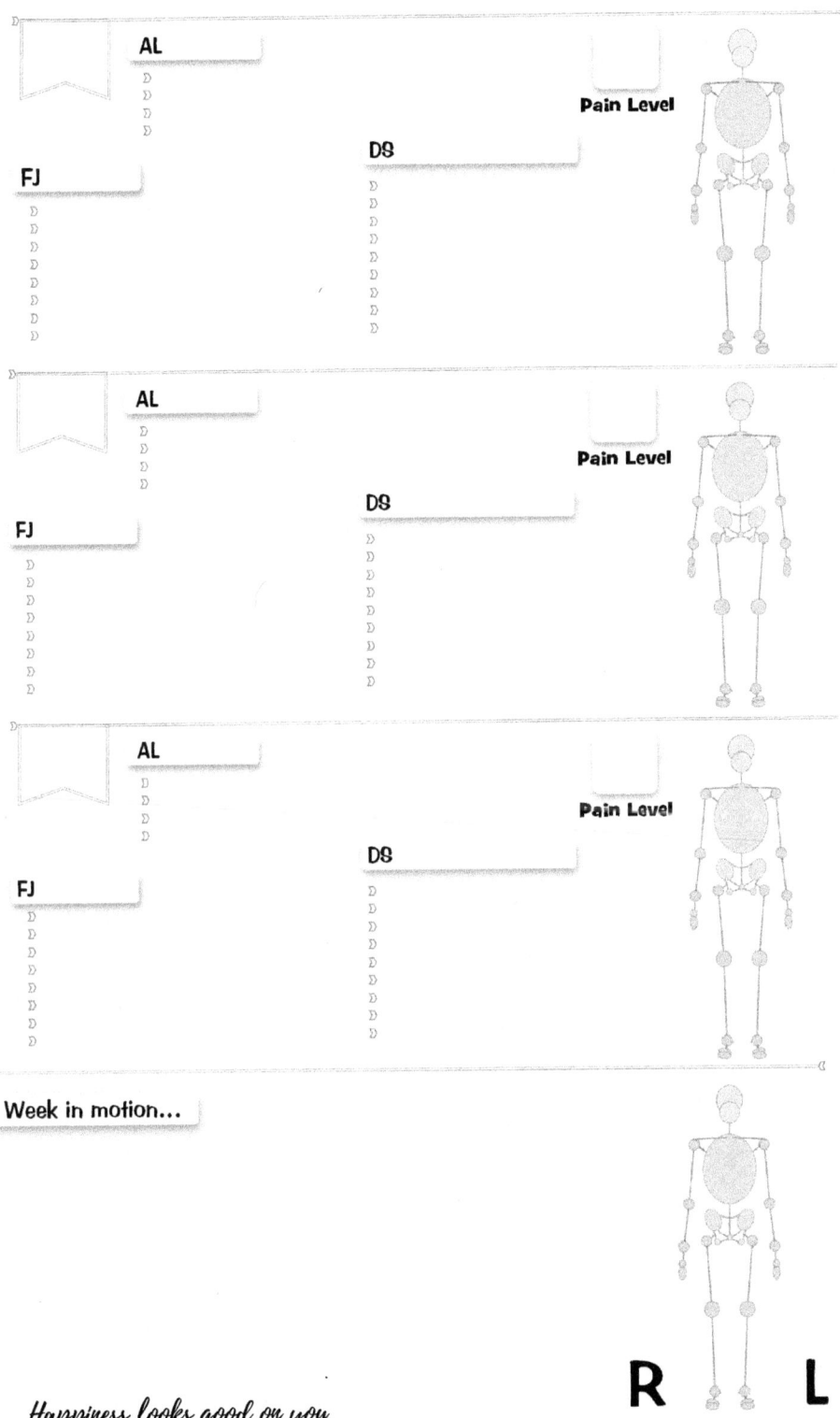

AL

- 〕
- 〕
- 〕
- 〕

Pain Level

FJ

- 〕
- 〕
- 〕
- 〕
- 〕
- 〕
- 〕

DS

- 〕
- 〕
- 〕
- 〕
- 〕
- 〕
- 〕

AL

- 〕
- 〕
- 〕
- 〕

Pain Level

FJ

- 〕
- 〕
- 〕
- 〕
- 〕
- 〕
- 〕

DS

- 〕
- 〕
- 〕
- 〕
- 〕
- 〕
- 〕

AL

- 〕
- 〕
- 〕
- 〕

Pain Level

FJ

- 〕
- 〕
- 〕
- 〕
- 〕
- 〕

DS

- 〕
- 〕
- 〕
- 〕
- 〕
- 〕
- 〕

Week in motion...

R   L

Happiness looks good on you.

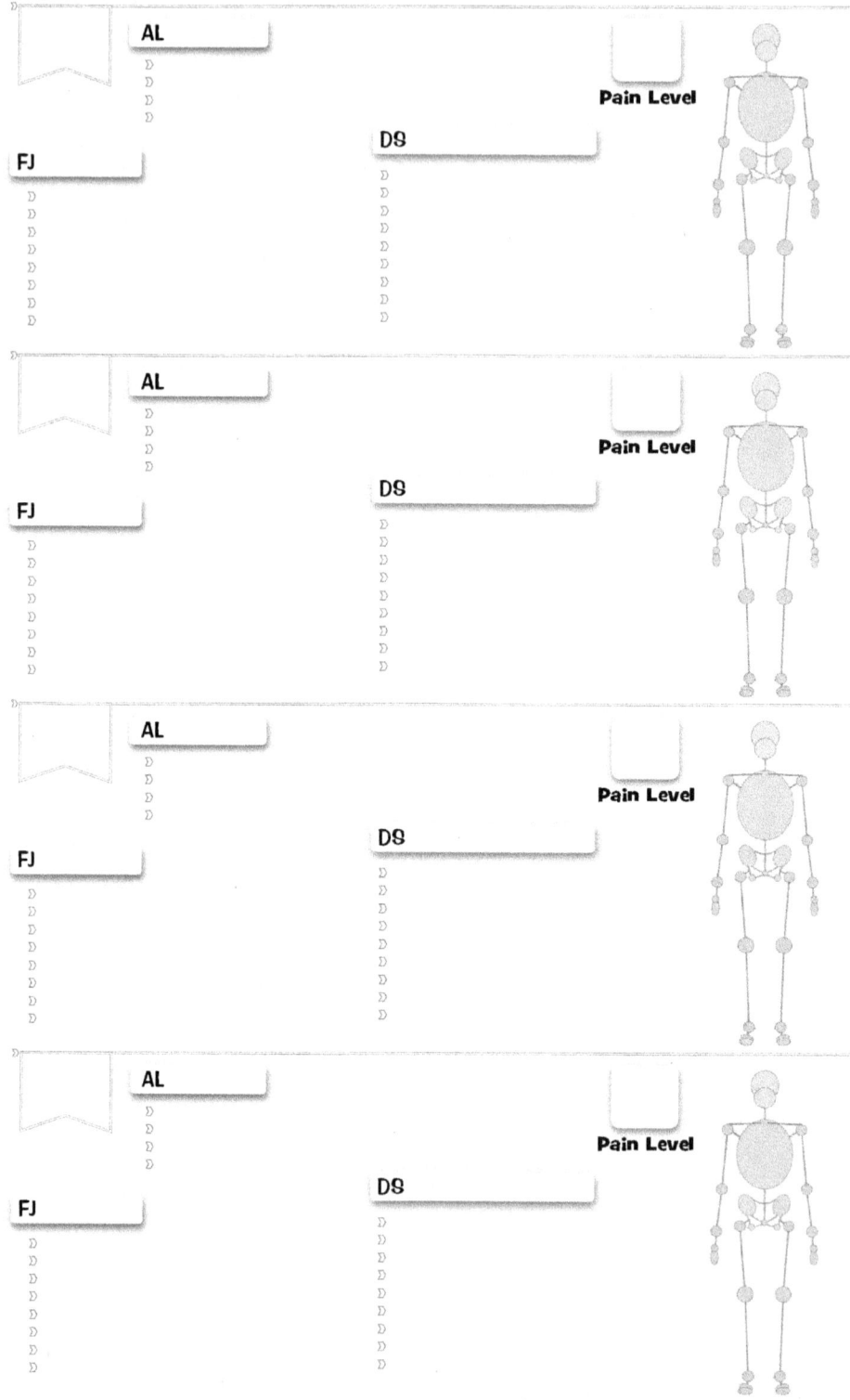

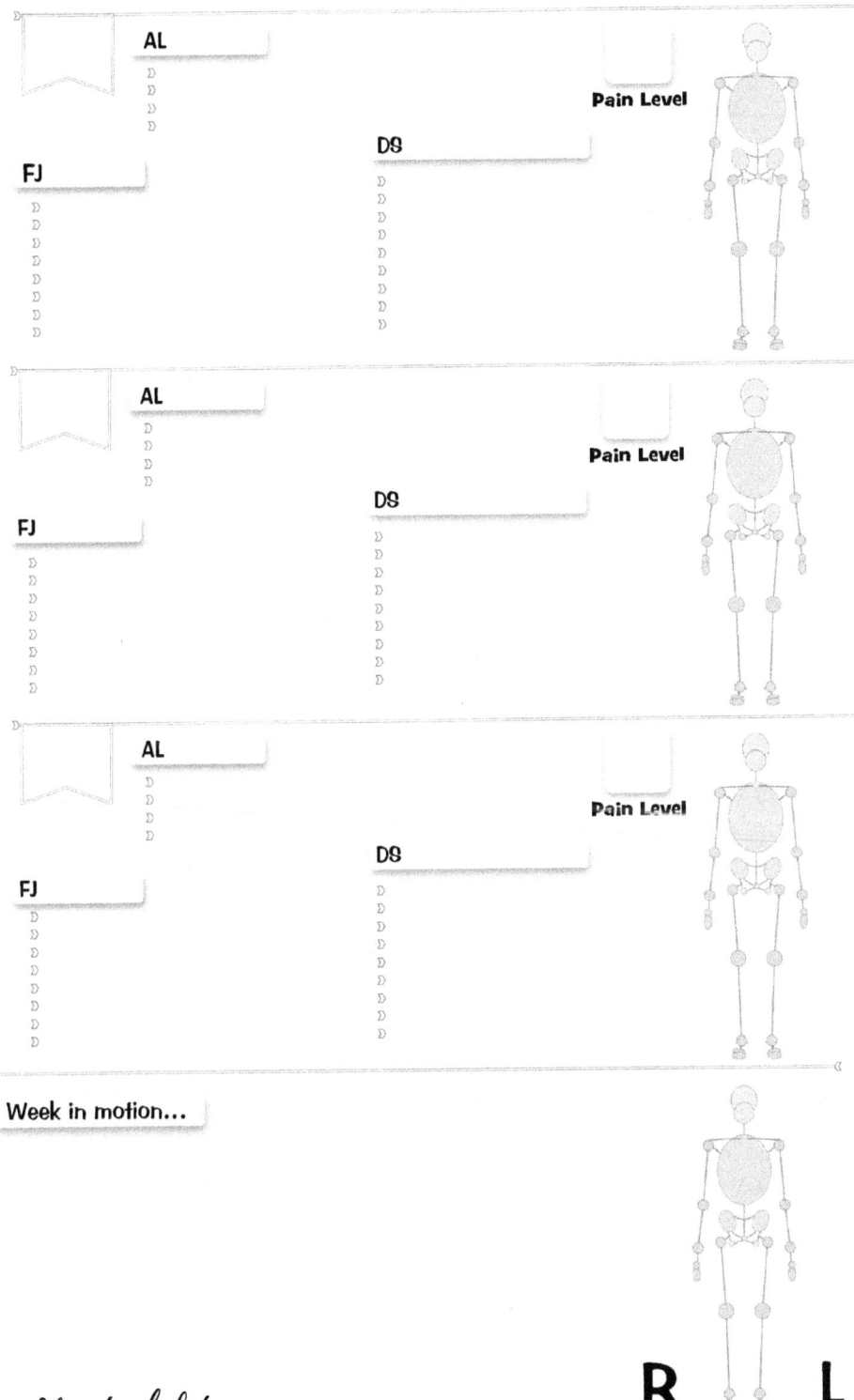

AL

FJ

DS

Pain Level

AL

FJ

DS

Pain Level

AL

FJ

DS

Pain Level

Week in motion...

Life is tough, but so are you. – UNK

R   L

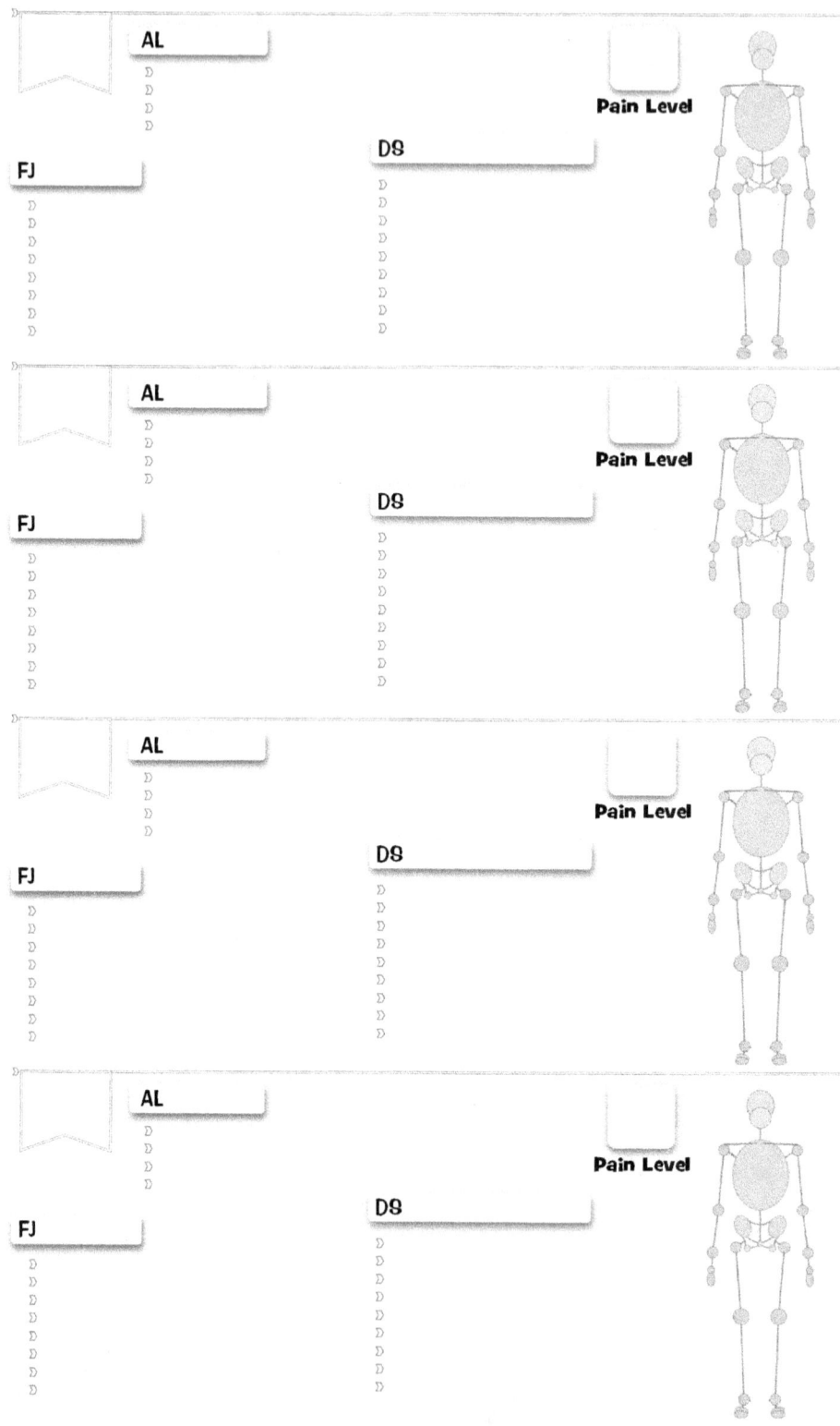

AL

FJ

DS

Pain Level

AL

FJ

DS

Pain Level

AL

FJ

DS

Pain Level

AL

FJ

DS

Pain Level

AL
D
D
D
D

Pain Level

FJ
D
D
D
D
D
D
D

DS
D
D
D
D
D
D
D

AL
D
D
D
D

Pain Level

FJ
D
D
D
D
D
D
D

DS
D
D
D
D
D
D
D

AL
D
D
D
D

Pain Level

FJ
D
D
D
D
D
D
D

DS
D
D
D
D
D
D
D

Week in motion...

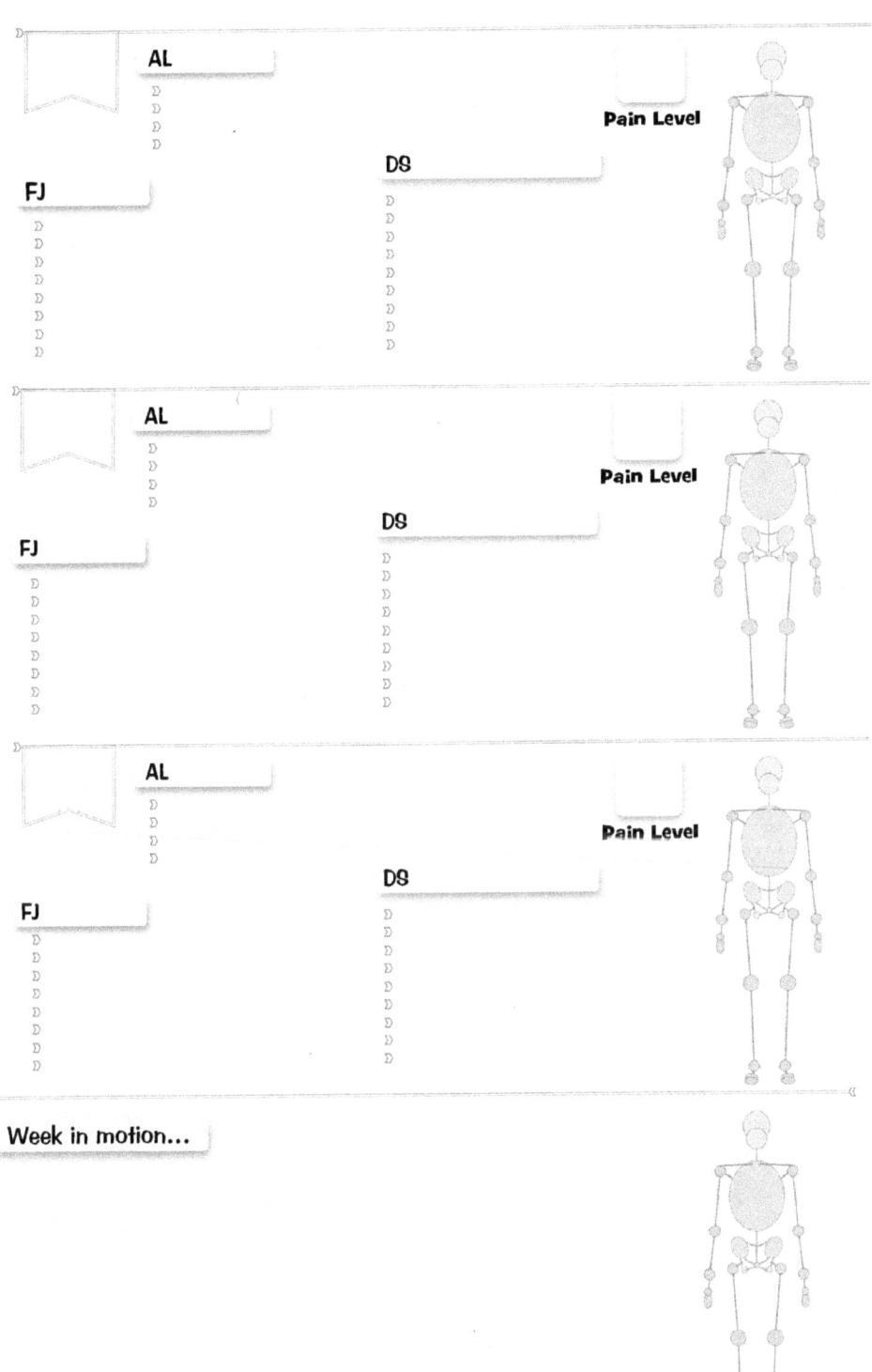

I'm pretty positive no good will come from focusing on the negative. – UNK

R   **L**

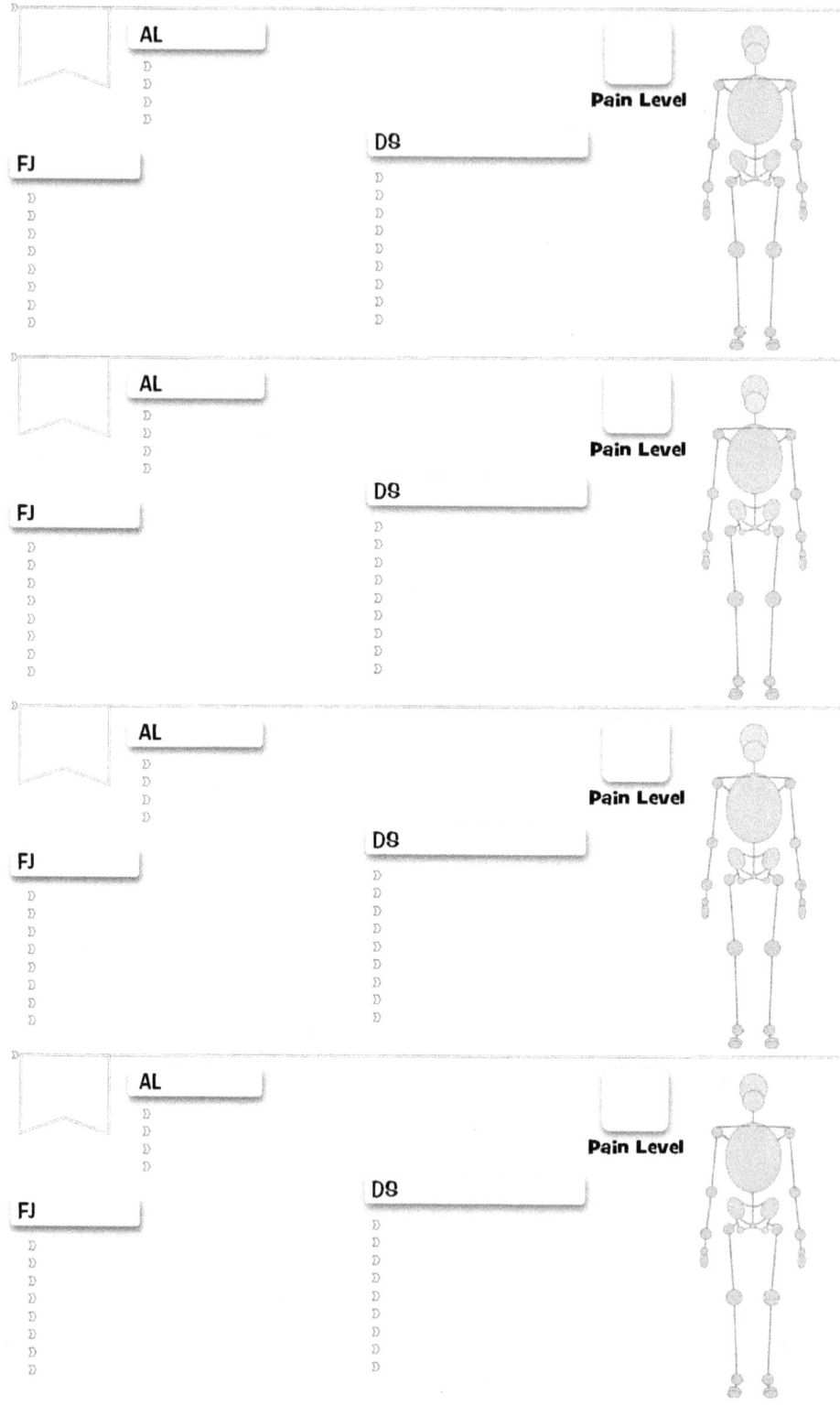

AL

FJ

DS

Pain Level

AL

FJ

DS

Pain Level

AL

FJ

DS

Pain Level

AL

FJ

DS

Pain Level

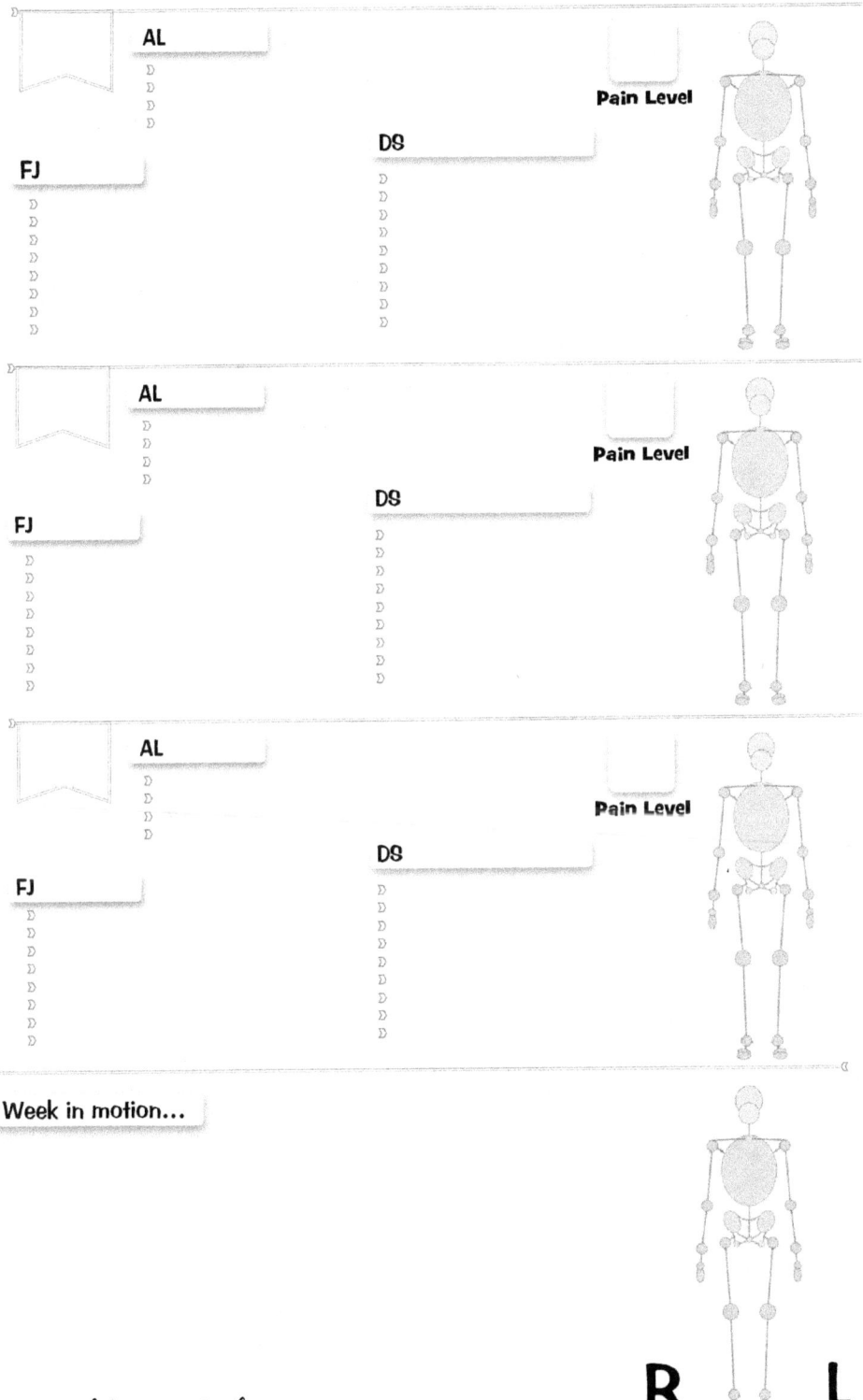

AL

FJ

DS

Pain Level

AL

FJ

DS

Pain Level

AL

FJ

DS

Pain Level

Week in motion...

R   L

Disability is not a bad word.

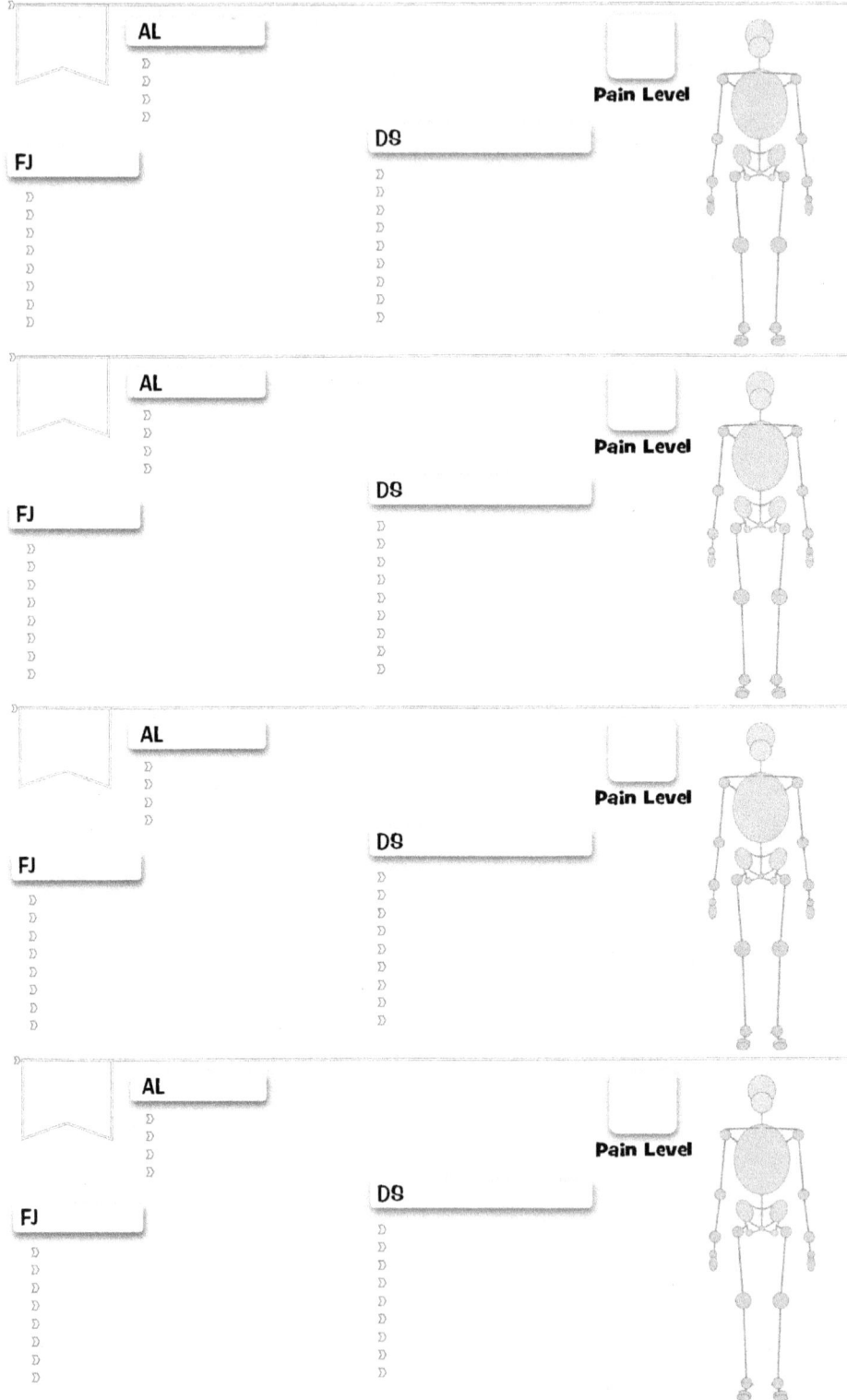

AL

FJ

Pain Level

DS

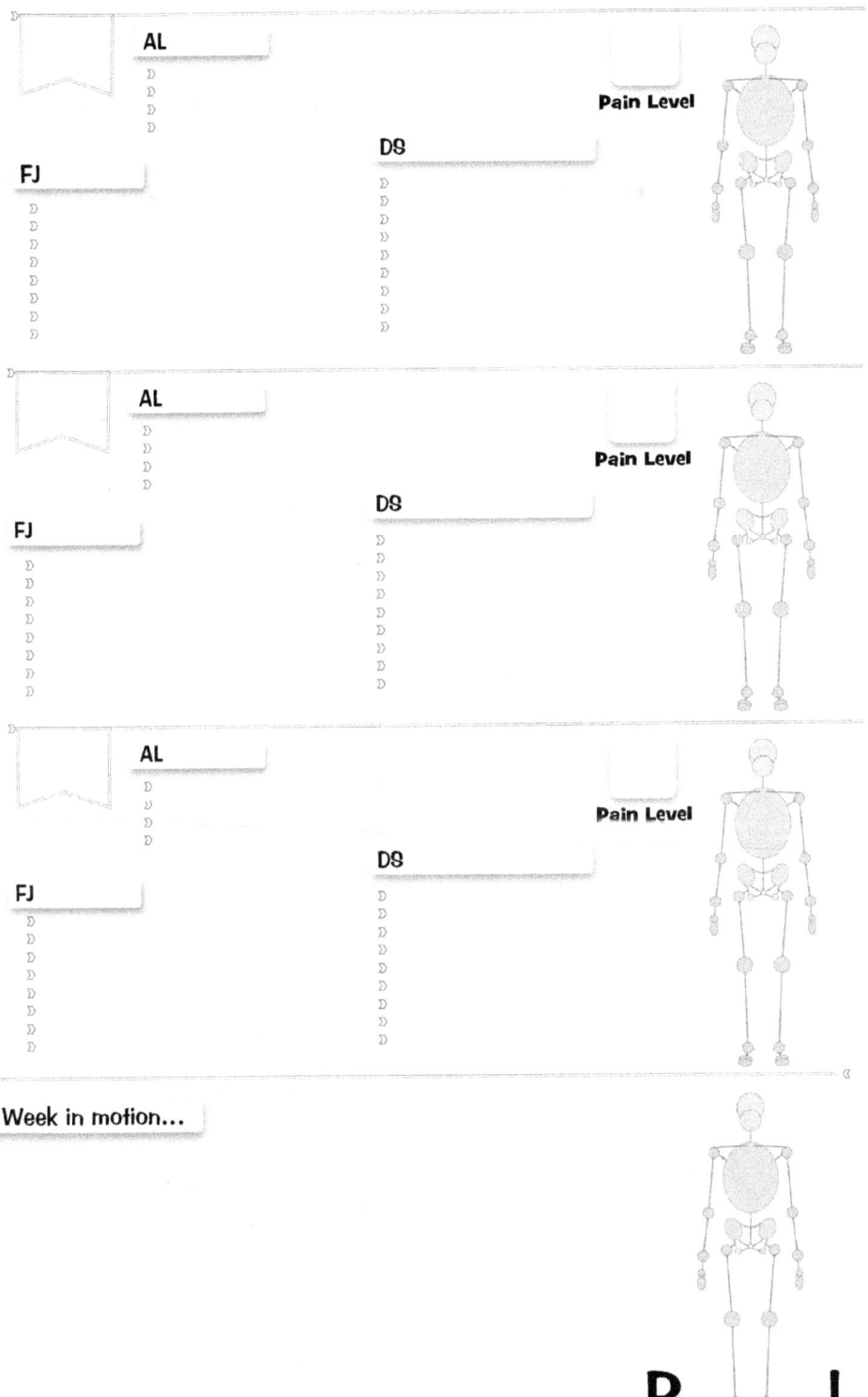

AL
- D
- D
- D
- D

FJ
- D
- D
- D
- D
- D
- D
- D

DS
- D
- D
- D
- D
- D
- D
- D

Pain Level

AL
- D
- D
- D
- D

FJ
- D
- D
- D
- D
- D
- D
- D

DS
- D
- D
- D
- D
- D
- D
- D

Pain Level

AL
- D
- D
- D
- D

FJ
- D
- D
- D
- D
- D
- D
- D

DS
- D
- D
- D
- D
- D
- D
- D

Pain Level

Week in motion...

R **L**

Don't tell people your dreams, show them. – UNK

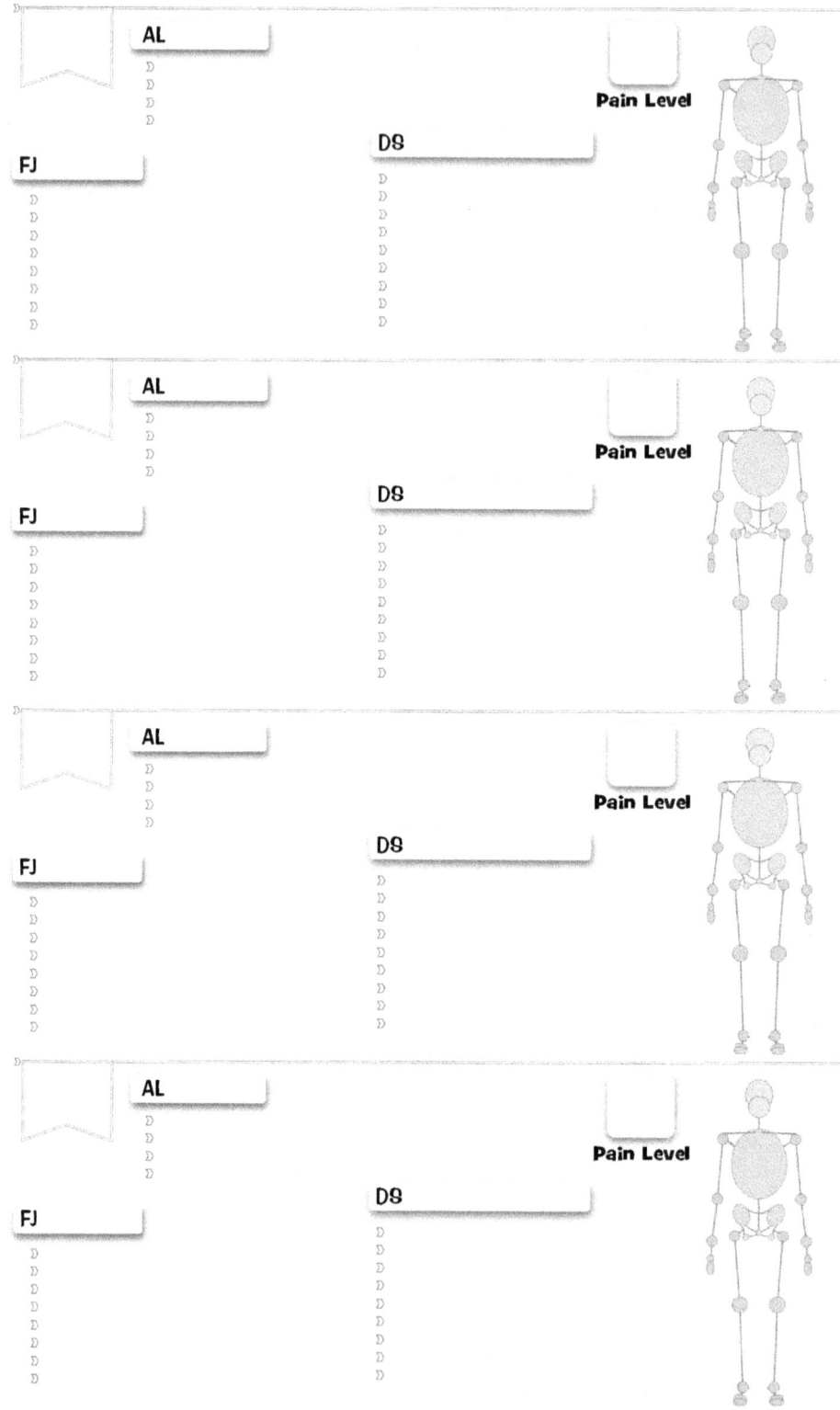

AL

FJ

DS

Pain Level

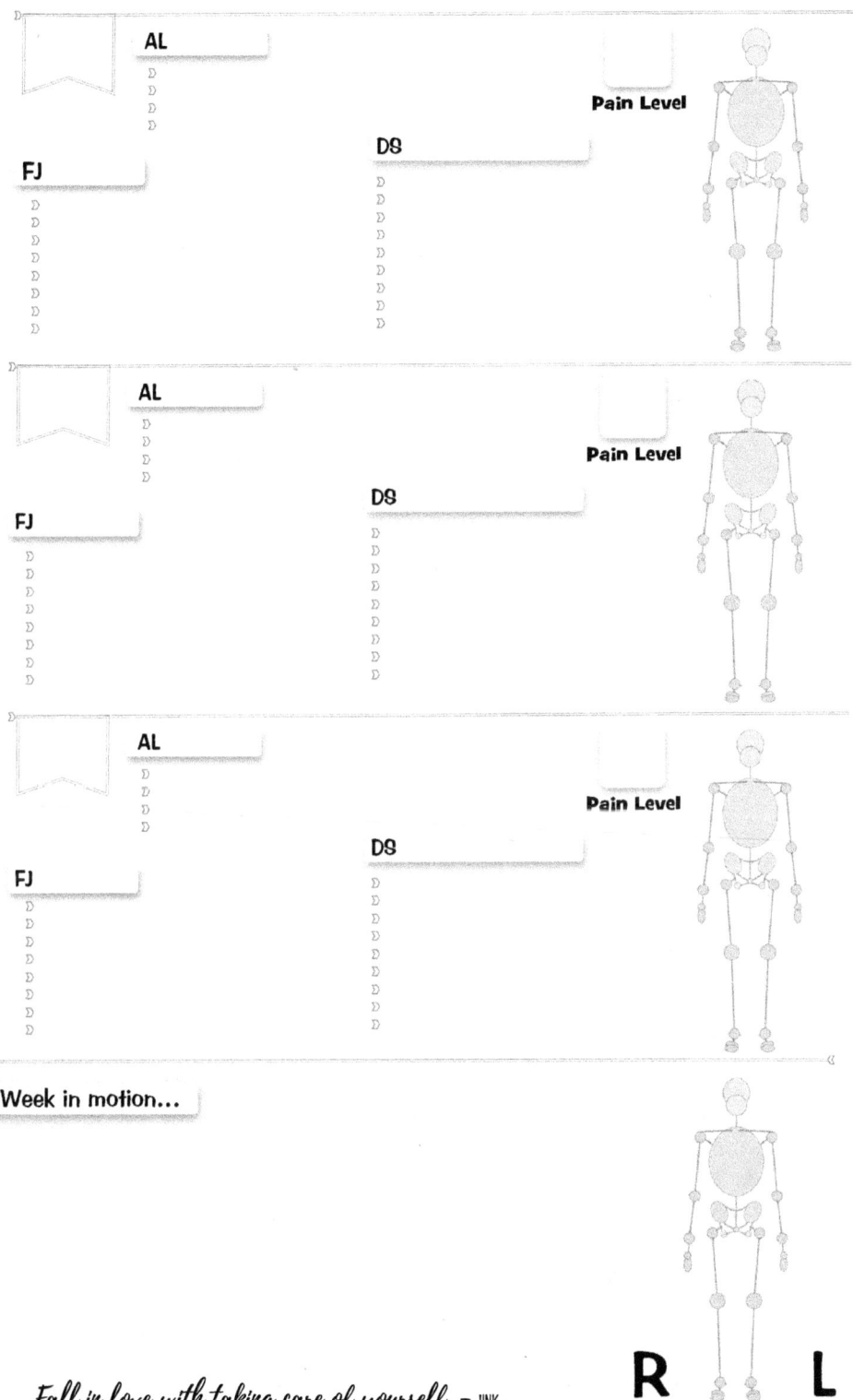

AL

FJ

DS

Pain Level

AL

FJ

DS

Pain Level

AL

FJ

DS

Pain Level

Week in motion...

R   L

Fall in love with taking care of yourself. – UNK

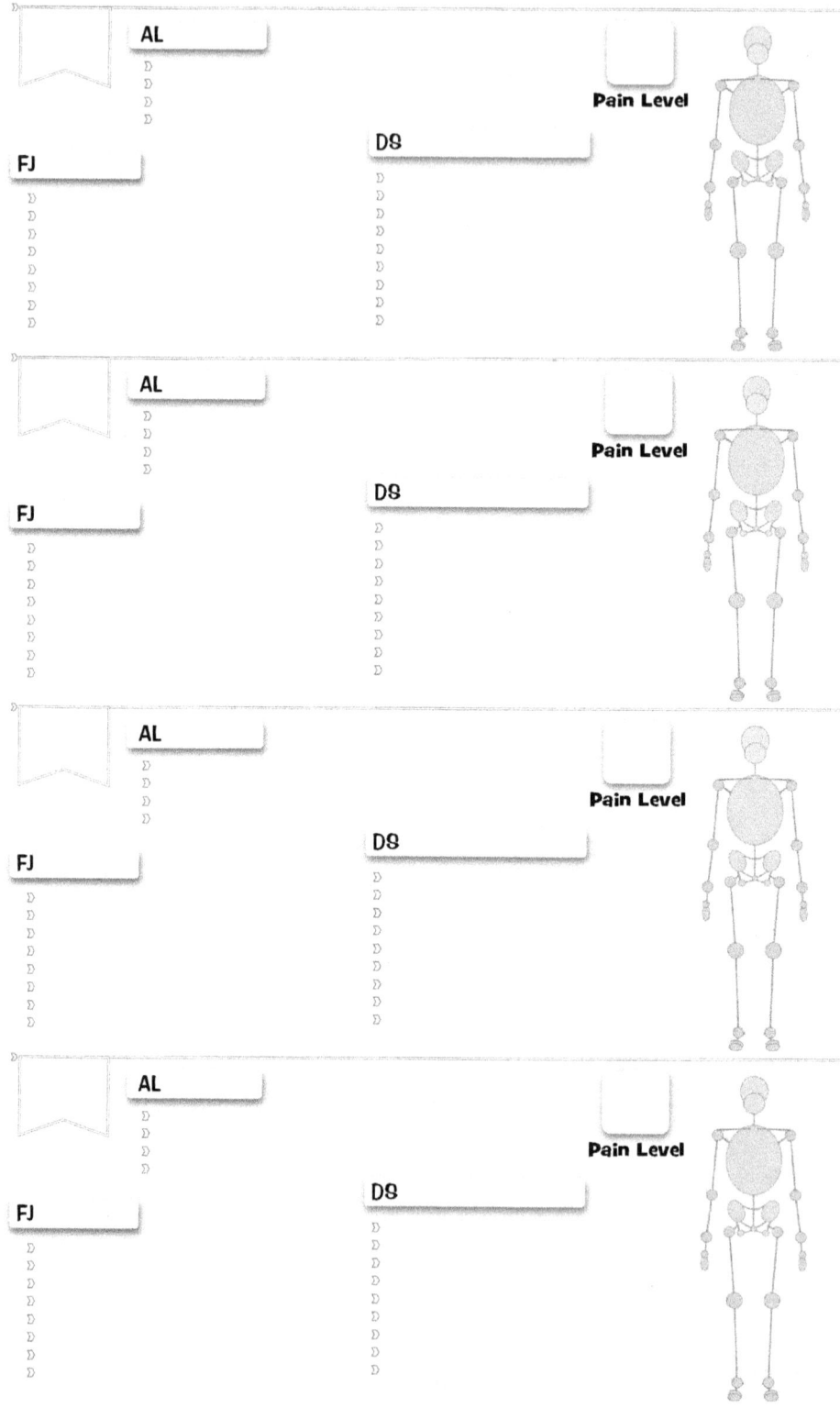

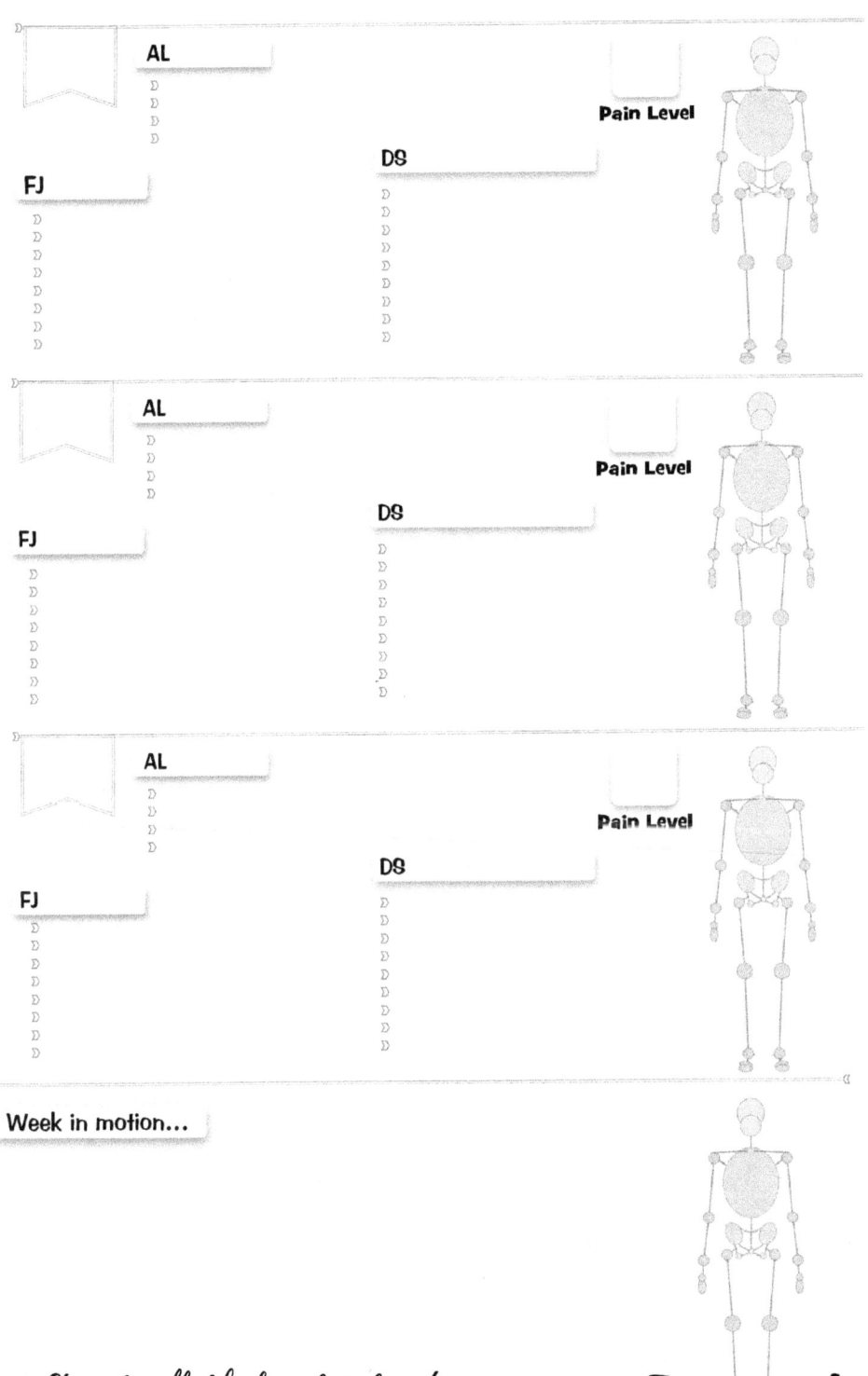

AL

Pain Level

DS

FJ

AL

Pain Level

DS

FJ

AL

Pain Level

DS

FJ

Week in motion...

Stressed spelled backwards is desserts.
Coincidence? I think not. – UNK

R L

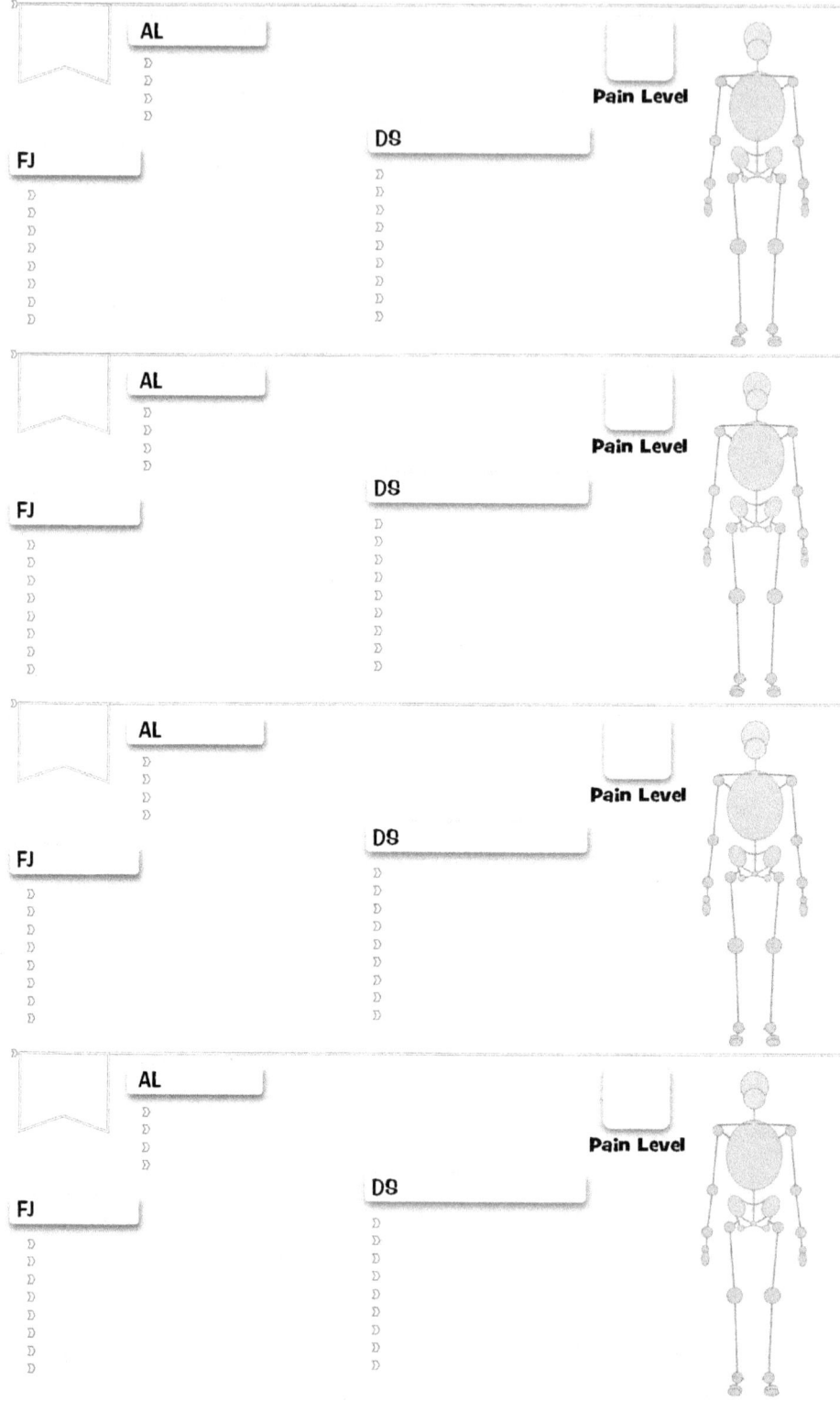

AL

FJ

DS

Pain Level

AL

FJ

DS

Pain Level

AL

FJ

DS

Pain Level

AL

FJ

DS

Pain Level

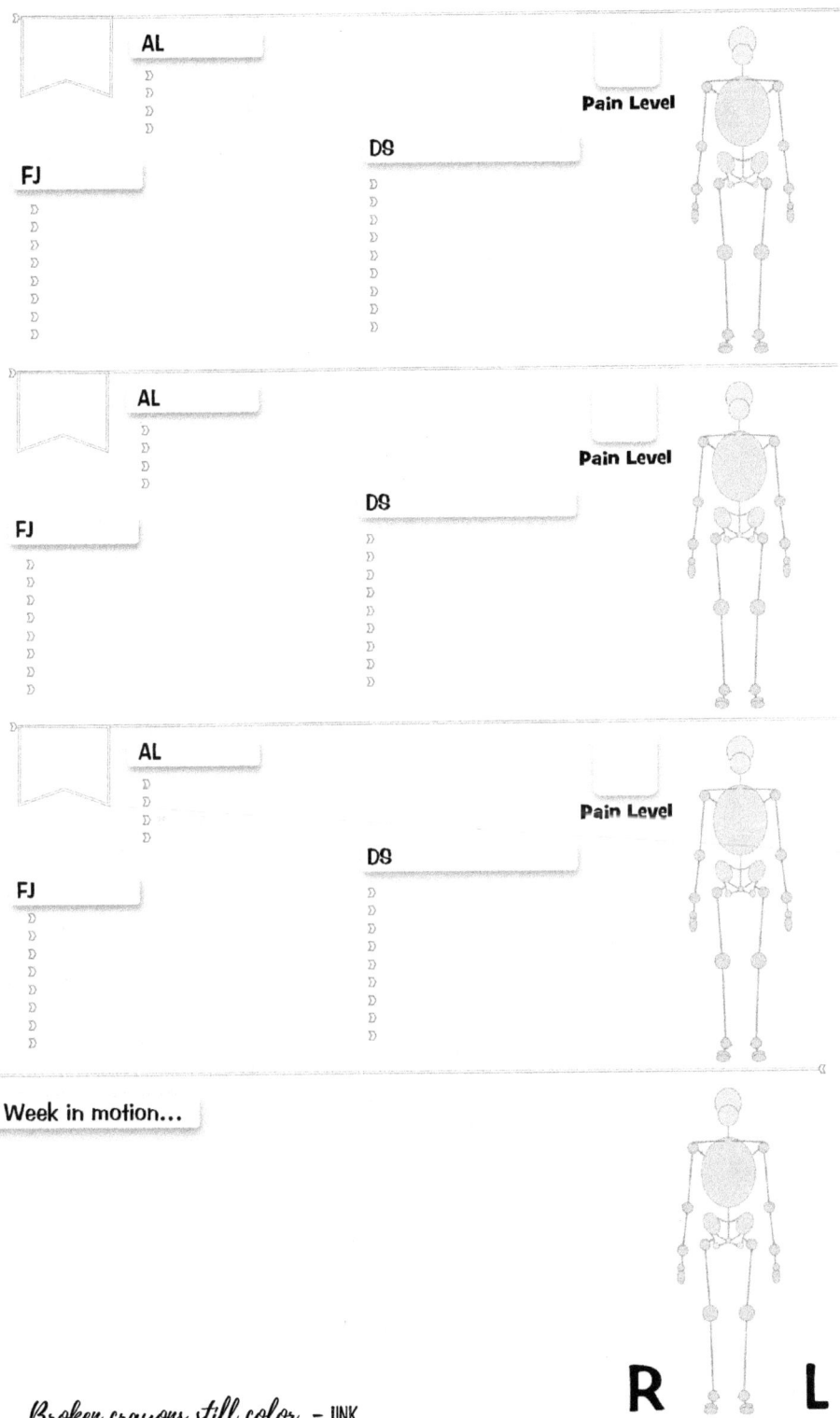

AL

FJ

DS

Pain Level

AL

FJ

DS

Pain Level

AL

FJ

DS

Pain Level

Week in motion...

R   **L**

Broken crayons still color. – UNK

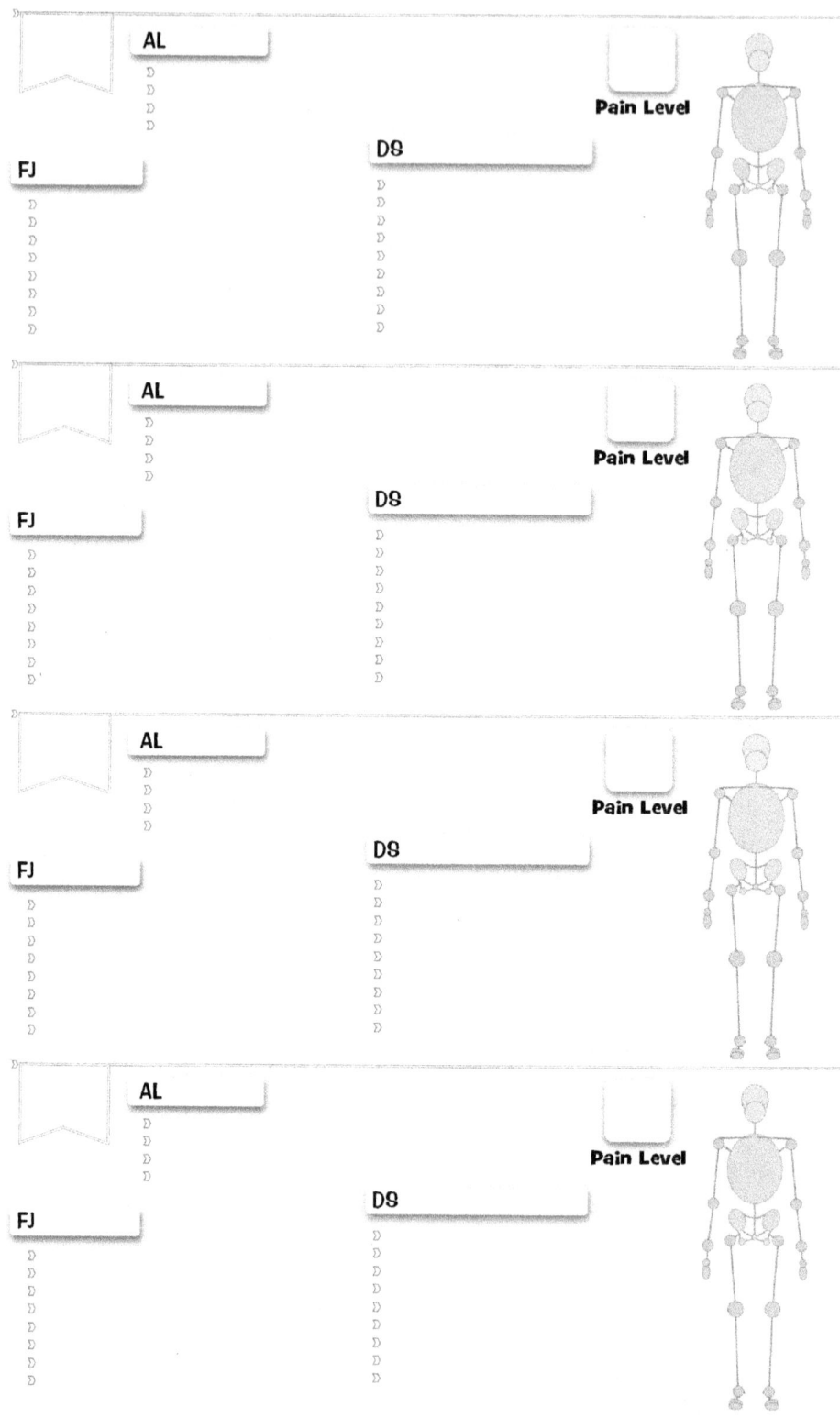

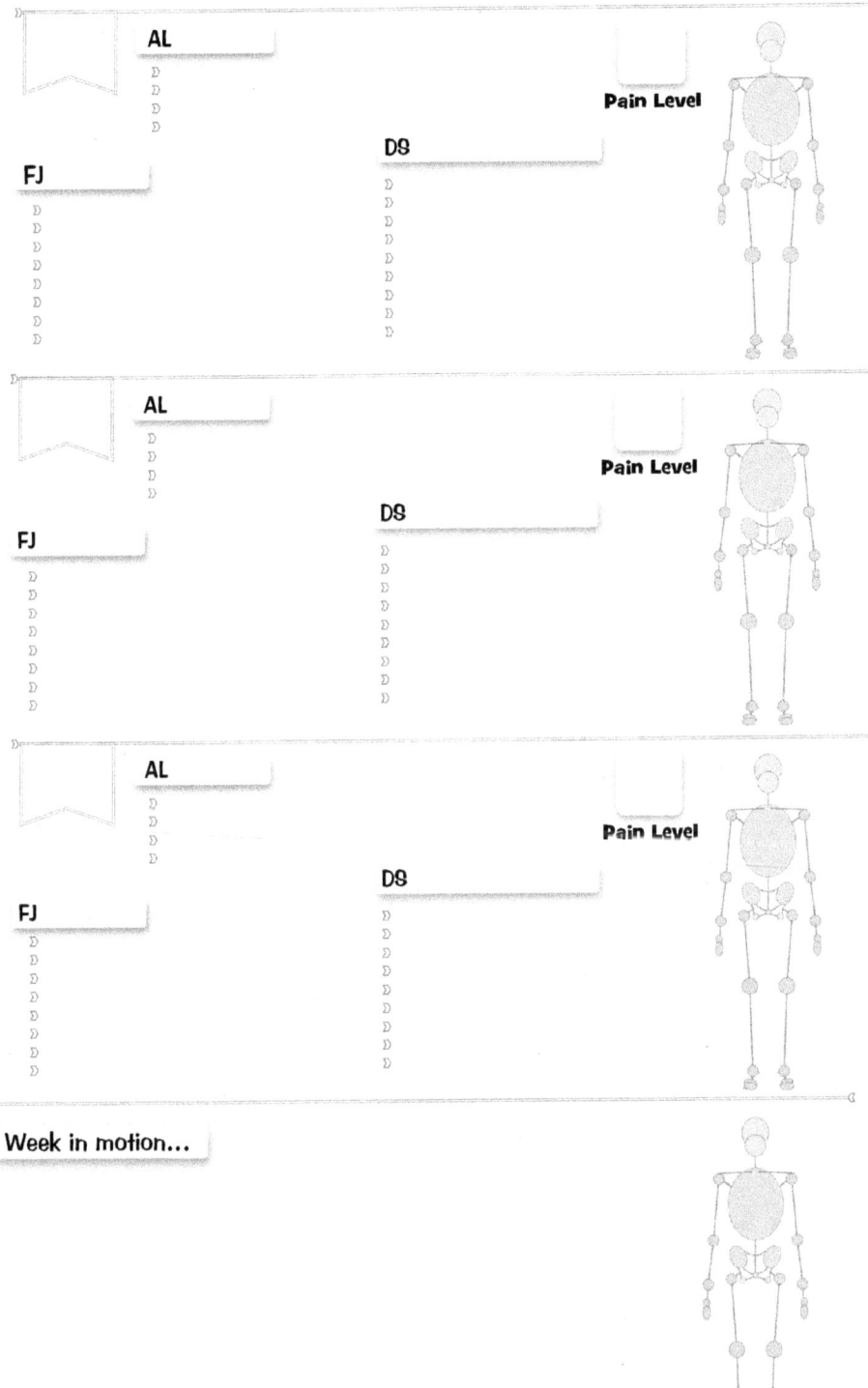

AL

> 》
> 》
> 》
> 》

Pain Level

FJ

> 》
> 》
> 》
> 》
> 》
> 》
> 》

DS

> 》
> 》
> 》
> 》
> 》
> 》
> 》

AL

> 》
> 》
> 》
> 》

Pain Level

FJ

> 》
> 》
> 》
> 》
> 》
> 》
> 》

DS

> 》
> 》
> 》
> 》
> 》
> 》
> 》

AL

> 》
> 》
> 》
> 》

Pain Level

FJ

> 》
> 》
> 》
> 》
> 》
> 》
> 》

DS

> 》
> 》
> 》
> 》
> 》
> 》
> 》

Week in motion...

We are all broken, that's how the light gets in. — ERNEST HEMINGWAY

R   **L**

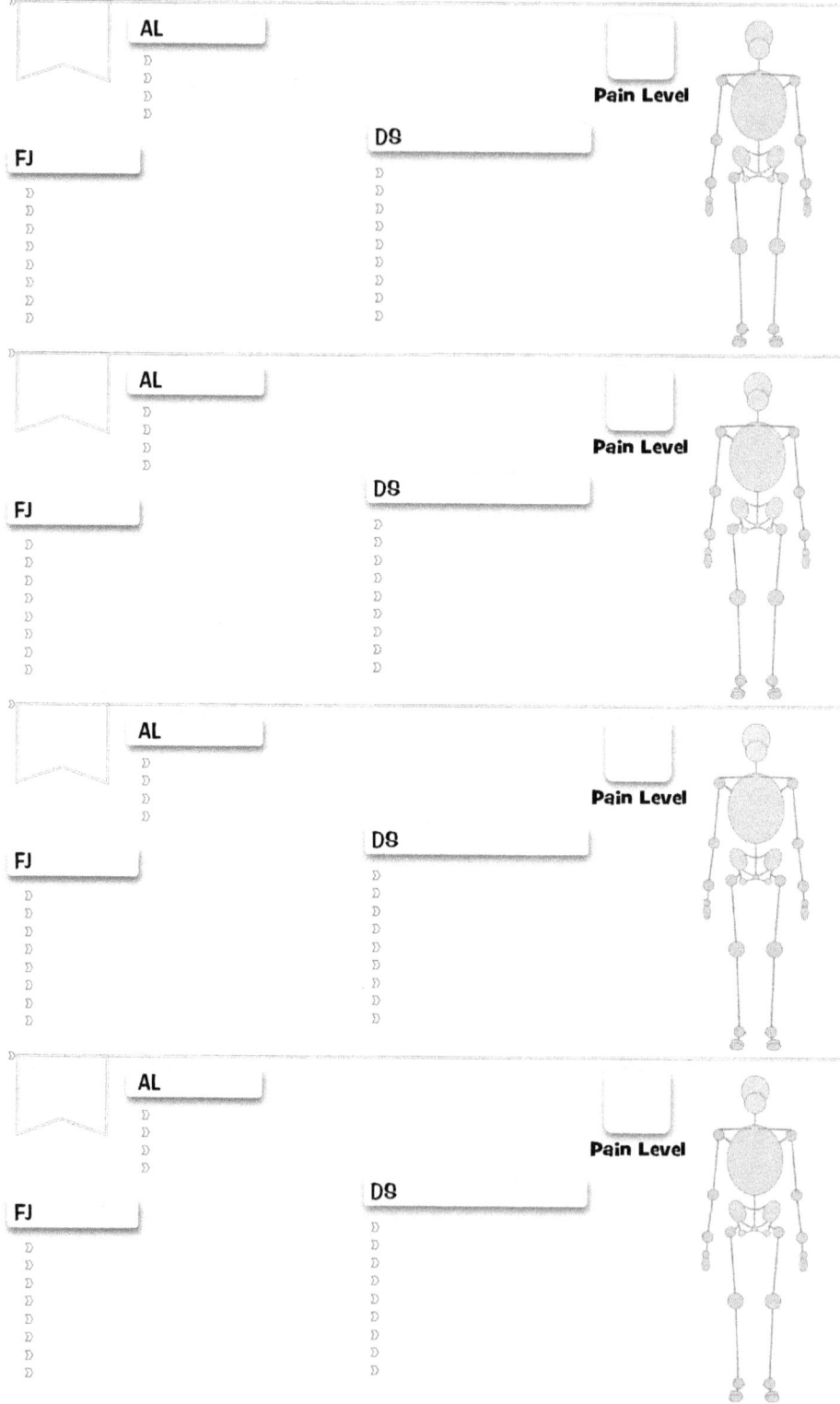

AL

FJ

DS

Pain Level

AL

FJ

DS

Pain Level

AL

FJ

DS

Pain Level

AL

FJ

DS

Pain Level

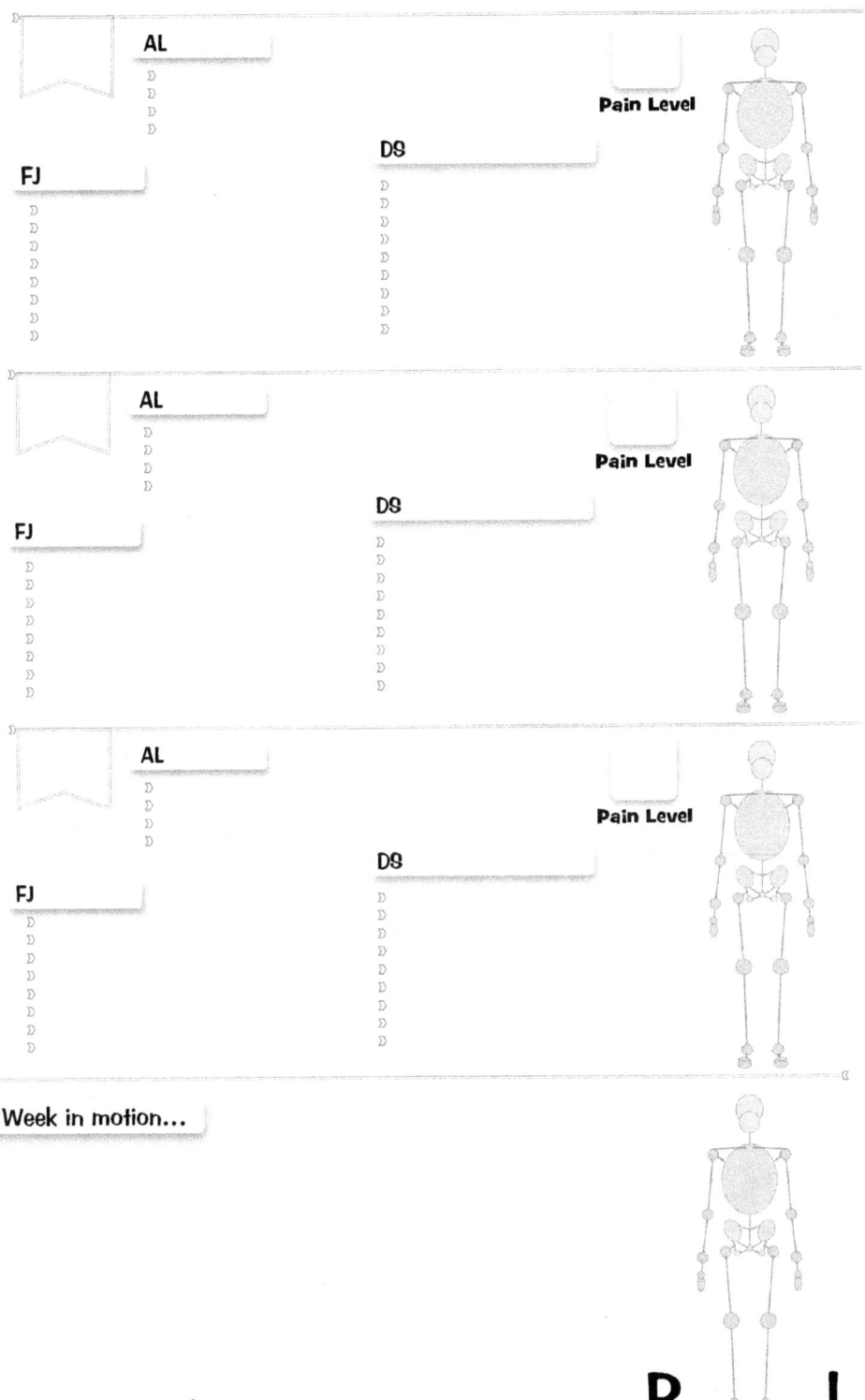

AL

> ⟩
> ⟩
> ⟩
> ⟩

Pain Level

DS

> ⟩
> ⟩
> ⟩
> ⟩
> ⟩
> ⟩
> ⟩

FJ

> ⟩
> ⟩
> ⟩
> ⟩
> ⟩
> ⟩
> ⟩

AL

> ⟩
> ⟩
> ⟩
> ⟩

Pain Level

DS

> ⟩
> ⟩
> ⟩
> ⟩
> ⟩
> ⟩
> ⟩

FJ

> ⟩
> ⟩
> ⟩
> ⟩
> ⟩
> ⟩
> ⟩

AL

> ⟩
> ⟩
> ⟩
> ⟩

Pain Level

DS

> ⟩
> ⟩
> ⟩
> ⟩
> ⟩
> ⟩
> ⟩

FJ

> ⟩
> ⟩
> ⟩
> ⟩
> ⟩
> ⟩
> ⟩

Week in motion...

R   **L**

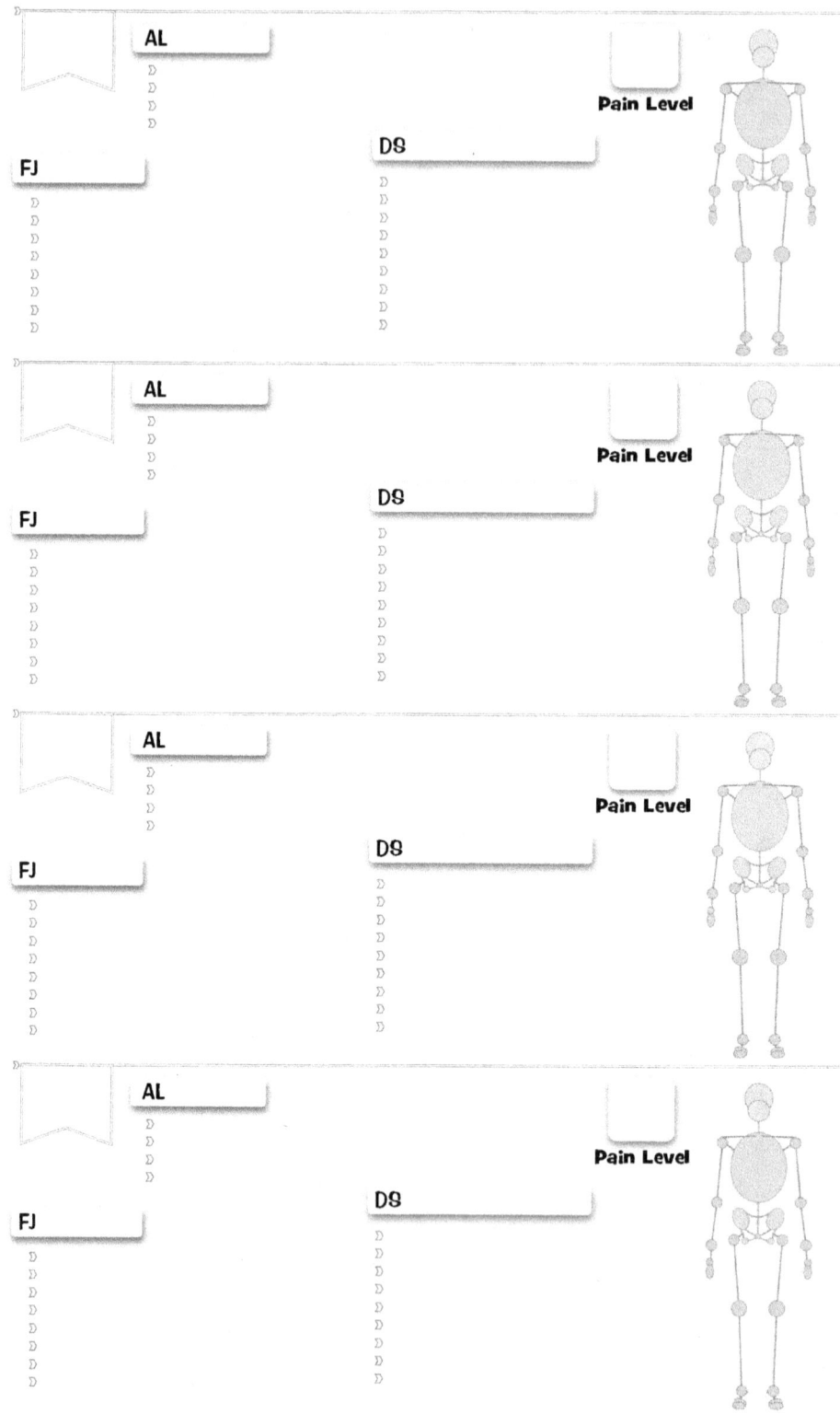

AL

FJ

DS

Pain Level

AL

Pain Level

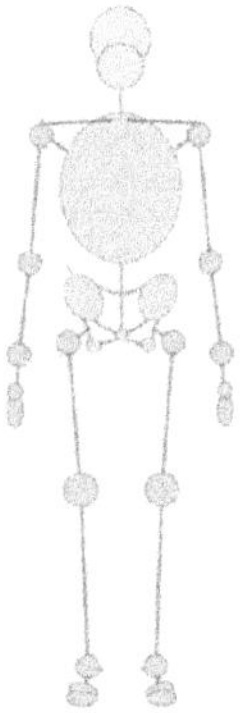

FJ

DS

AL

Pain Level

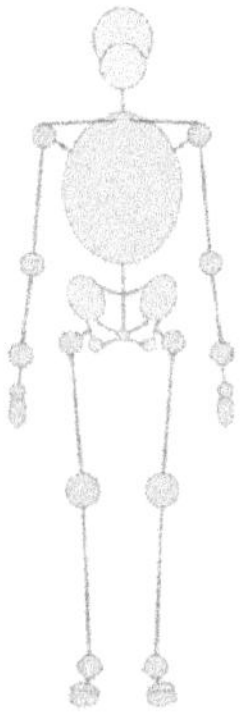

FJ

DS

AL

Pain Level

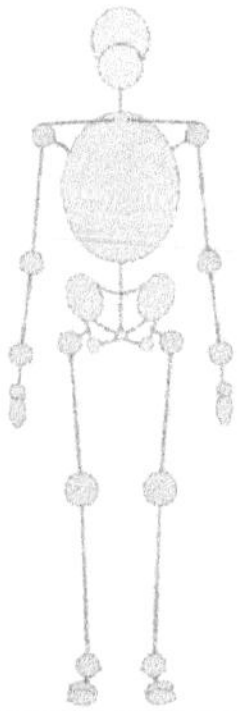

FJ

DS

Week in motion...

*Everything these days is about go go go but,
sometimes, what we need, is a bit more slow slow slow.* – UNK

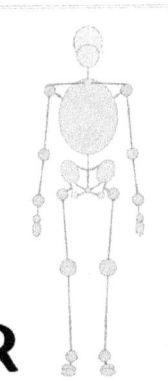

R   L

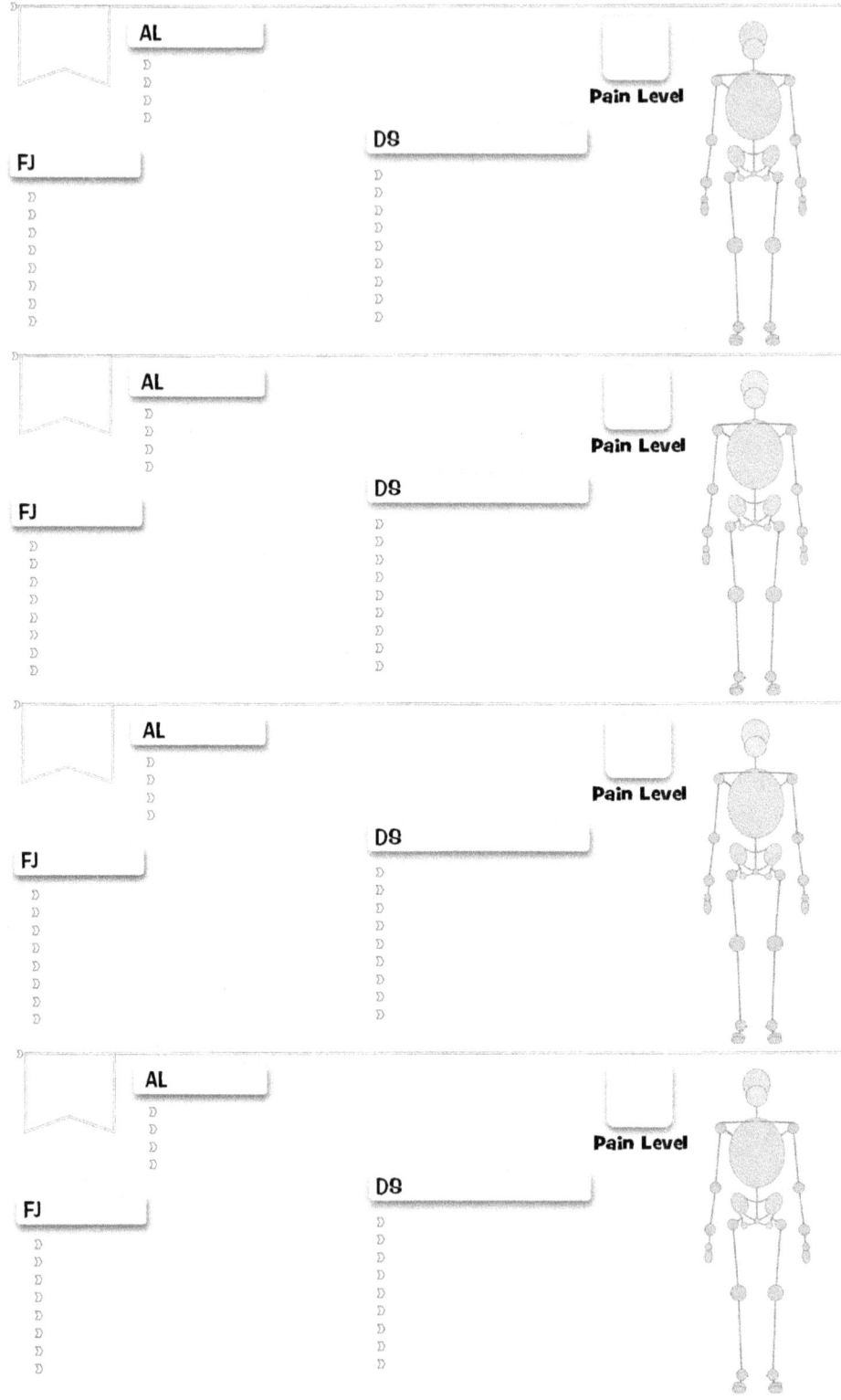

AL

Pain Level

FJ

DS

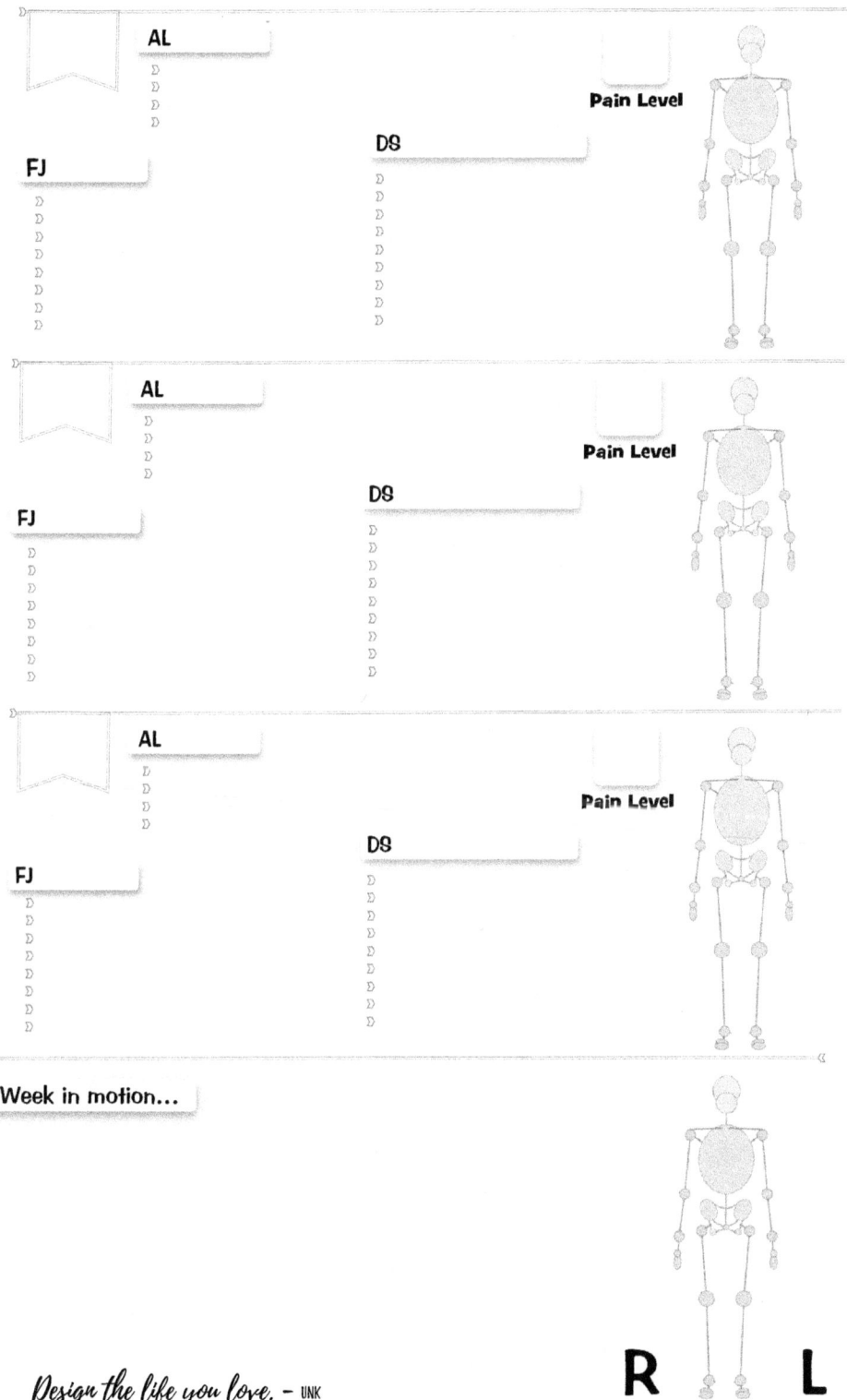

AL

FJ

DS

Pain Level

AL

FJ

DS

Pain Level

AL

FJ

DS

Pain Level

Week in motion...

R   L

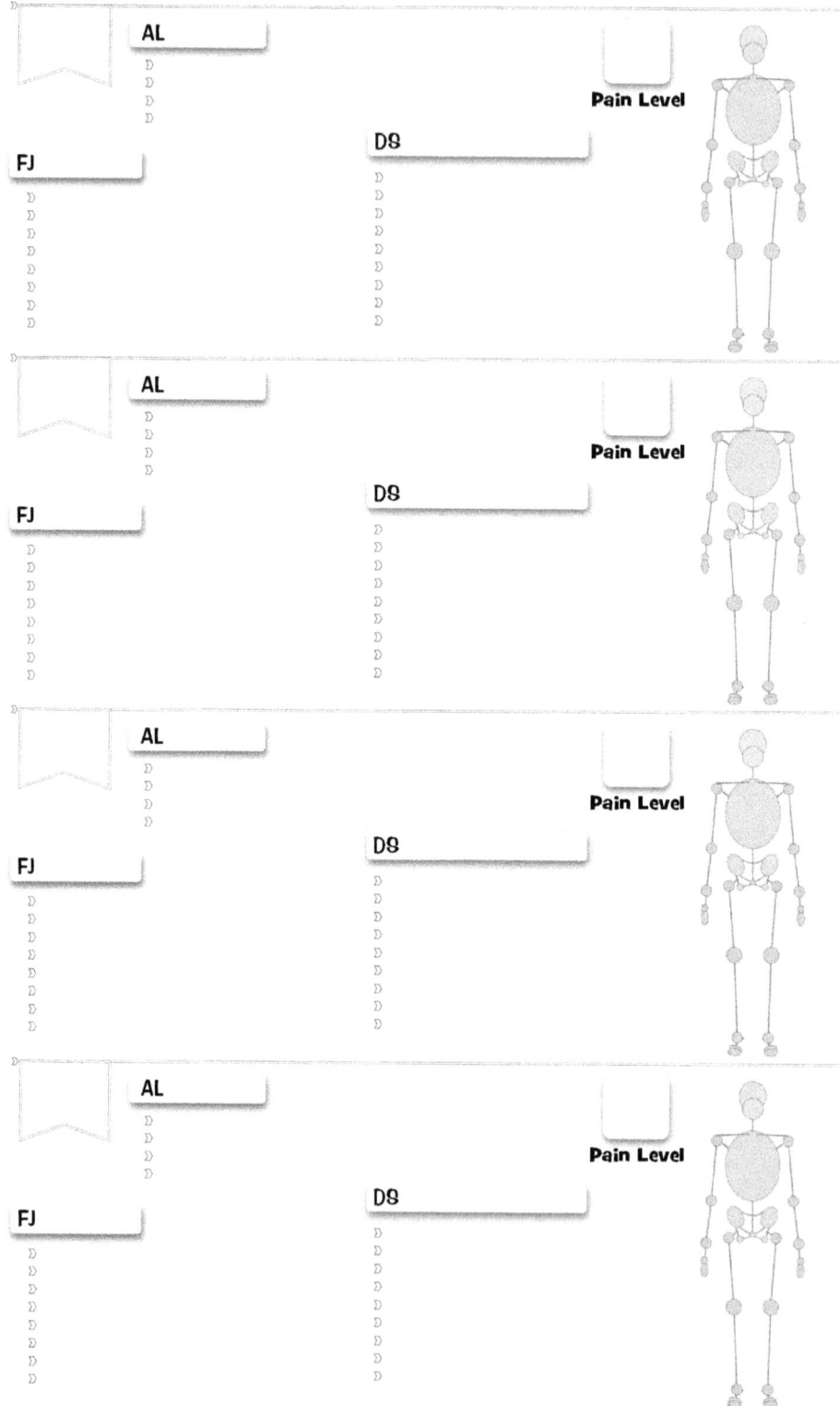

AL

FJ

DS

Pain Level

AL

FJ

DS

Pain Level

AL

FJ

DS

Pain Level

AL

FJ

DS

Pain Level

AL

FJ

DS

Pain Level

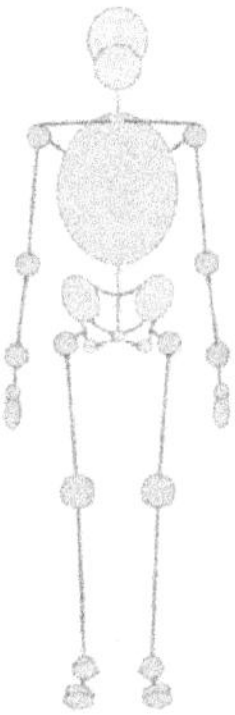

AL

FJ

DS

Pain Level

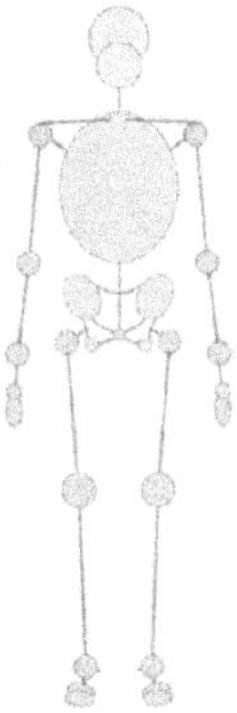

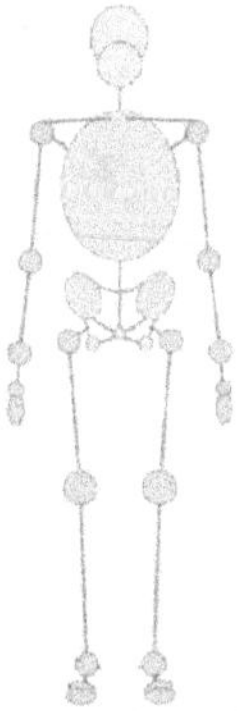

AL

FJ

DS

Pain Level

Week in motion...

If you ever find yourself feeling useless, remember that your breath provides carbon dioxide for plants and trees to thrive. – UNK

R 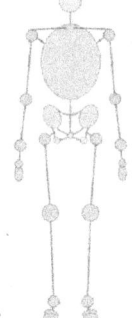 **L**

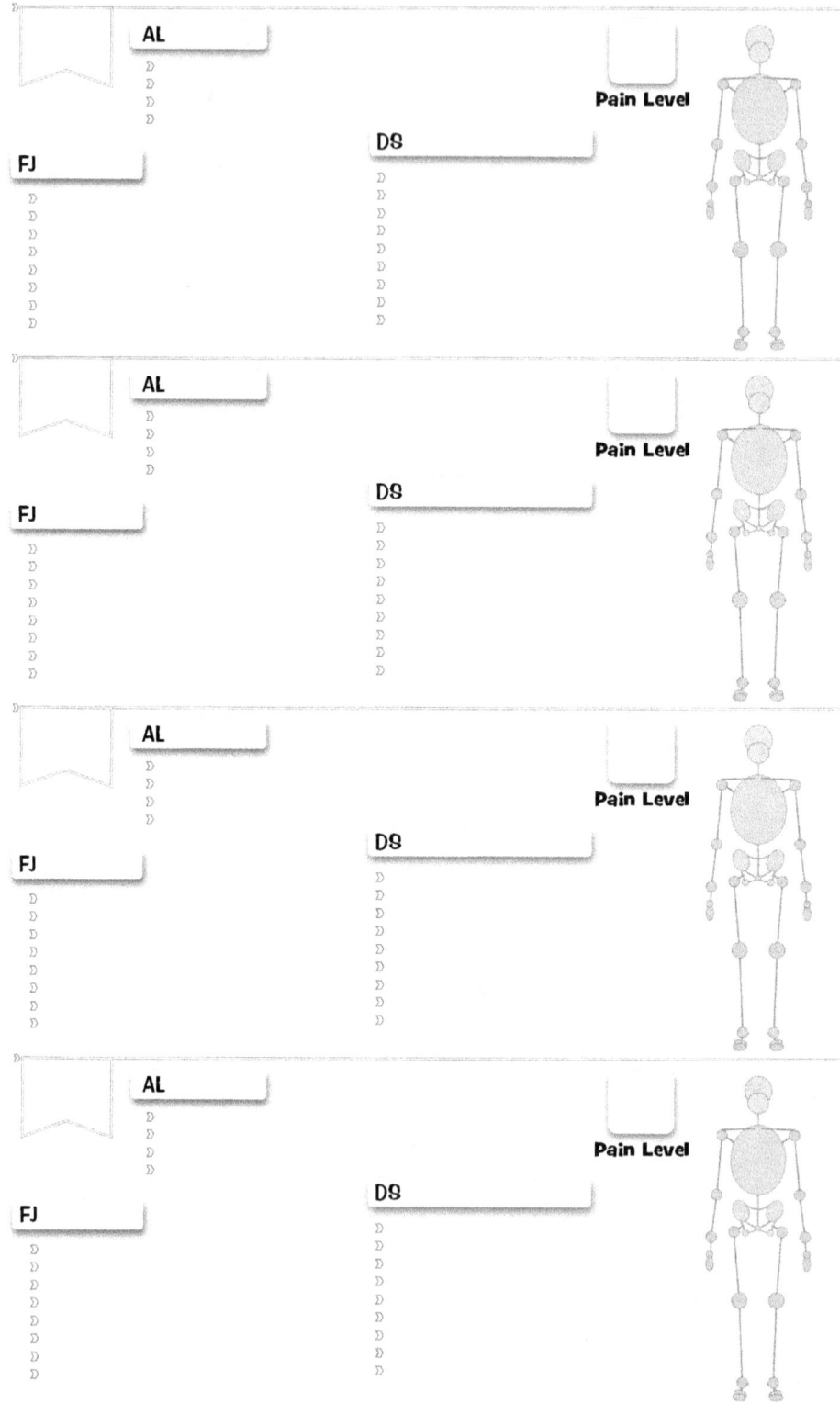

AL

FJ

DS

Pain Level

AL

FJ

DS

Pain Level

AL

FJ

DS

Pain Level

AL

FJ

DS

Pain Level

AL
- D
- D
- D

Pain Level

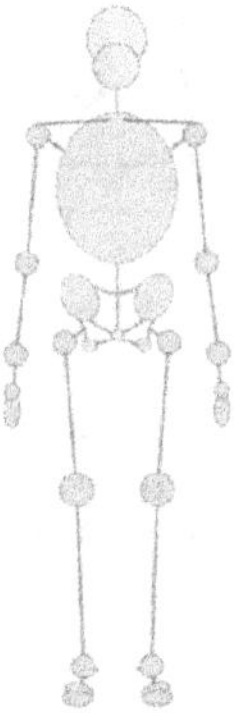

FJ
- D
- D
- D
- D
- D
- D
- D

DS
- D
- D
- D
- D
- D
- D
- D

AL
- D
- D
- D

Pain Level

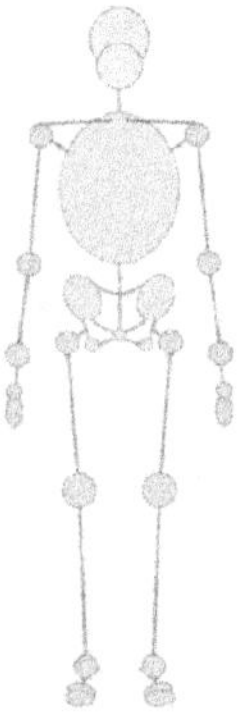

FJ
- D
- D
- D
- D
- D
- D
- D

DS
- D
- D
- D
- D
- D
- D
- D

AL
- D
- D
- D

Pain Level

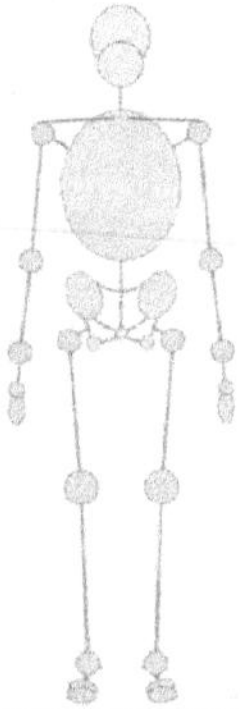

FJ
- D
- D
- D
- D
- D
- D
- D

DS
- D
- D
- D
- D
- D
- D
- D

Week in motion...

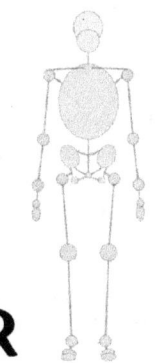

It's always a good time to let go of whatever is holding you back. — DANIELLE LA PORTE

R   L

GLOSSARY

Ehlers-Danlos syndrome as defined by the Genetics Home reference website
"Ehlers-Danlos syndrome is a group of disorders that affect the connective tissues
that support the skin, bones, blood vessels, and many other organs and tissues.
Defects in connective tissues cause the signs and symptoms of Ehlers-Danlos
syndrome, which vary from mildly loose joints to life-threatening complications."
https://ghr.nlm.nih.gov/condition/ehlers-danlos-syndrome#resources

The following terms are largely associated with the Ehlers-Danlos syndromes and its known
comorbidities. If you have any questions regarding and of these terms, or EDS
please consult your caregiver.

- Cellular - If you have excessive and/or frequent allergic reactions or anaphylactic episodes. These symptoms can be handled by immunologists, allergists, or other specialists.
- Cardiovascular - Any symptoms that involve blood pressure/heart rate regulation. These symptoms are usually managed by cardiologists, or other autonomic specialists.
- Orthopaedic - Conditions involving the musculoskeletal system. These symptoms are managed by orthopedists, podiatrists, or other specialists.
- Gastrointestinal - Relating to the stomach and intestines. These symptoms are largely managed by Gastroenterologists.
- Psychiatric - Related to mood, perceptual, and cognitive behaviors. These symptoms are managed by psychiatrists, and therapists.
- Oral/Mandibular - Of or relating to the mouth, mandible, and the temporomandibular joint (TMJ). These symptoms are managed by Dentists, and other specialists.
- Neuro - Relating to the nerves or nervous system. These symptoms can be managed by neurologists, physical medicine specialist or other related specialists.
- Spinal - Relating to the spine. These symptoms can be managed by varying specialists.

- Acute Pain - Any type of pain that lasts less than 3 - 6 months, or pain that is directly related to soft tissue damage.
- Anaphylaxis - A severe and potentially life-threatening allergic reaction.
- Angioedema - An area of severe swelling just under the skin.
- Atlantoaxial Instability - Abnormal movement in the neck between the first and second vertebrae.
- Chiari I Malformation - CMI - A condition in which the brain tissue extends into the spinal canal.
- Chronic Pain - Any type of pain that persists longer than 3 - 6 months.
- Connective Tissue - Tissue that connects, binds, or separates other tissues or organs (bone/cartilage/blood/fat).
- Craniocervical Instability - CCI - The structural instability of the craniocervical joints.
- Dysmotility - A condition in which the muscles of the digestive system become impaired and changes in speed, strength or coordination.
- Dystonia - Involuntary muscle contractions.
- Heritable - A biologic transmission from parent to offspring.

- Hypermobility - An increased range of motion of a joint or body part, beyond the normal range.
- Instability - A lack of stability.
- Idiopathic - Any condition that arises spontaneously or for which the cause is unknown.
- Idiopathic Intracranial Hypertension - IIH
  Intracranial hypertension is a condition due to high pressure within the spaces that surround the brain and spinal cord. These spaces are filled with cerebrospinal fluid (CSF), which cushions the brain from mechanical injury, provides nourishment, and carries away waste. [1]
- Mandible - Jaw, or a jawbone. Usually the lower jawbone in mammals and fishes. Largest bone in the face.
- MCAS/MCAD - Mast Cell Activation Disorder/Mast Cell Activation Syndrome.
- Musculoskeletal system - Involving the joints, ligament, muscles, nerves, tendons, and structures that support the limbs, neck and back.
- Neurally Mediated Hypotension - NMH - Neurally mediated syncope is a disorder of the autonomic regulation of postural tone, which results in hypotension, bradycardia, and loss of consciousness. [2]
- Orthostatic Hypotension - OH True orthostatic hypotension (OH) was defined by consensus in 2011 as sustained reduction of systolic BP >20 mm Hg or of diastolic BP >10 mm Hg within 3 minutes of standing or head-up tilt. [3]
- Orthostatic Intolerance - "Loss of consciousness or lesser cognitive deficits (memory loss, decreased reasoning and concentration), visual difficulties, lightheadedness, headache, fatigue, either increases (hypertension) or decreases (hypotension) of BP, weakness, nausea and abdominal pain, sweating, tremulousness, and exercise intolerance. [4]
- Pacing - The act or process of regulating or changing the timing of movement and activities to prolong your physical ability to perform said actions.
- Peri-operative anaphylaxis - Anaphylaxis during anesthesia.
- Peripheral Neuropathy - Weakness, numbness and pain from nerve damage (usually in the hands and feet).
- POTS - POTS is defined by chronic day-to-day symptoms of OI plus excessive increase in HR when upright. [5]
- Prolapse - A slipping (forward or down) of one of the parts of organs in the body.
- Proprioception - the sense of the relative position of one's own parts of the body and strength of effort being employed in movement.
- Pruritis - An unpleasant sensation that provokes the urge to scratch (can occur on any part of the body).
- Rhinitis - Most commonly referred to as seasonal allergies causing itchy/watery eyes, sneezing and other allergic symptoms.
- Segmental Kyphosis - An exaggerated curve of the thoracic spine.
- Skin flushing - Feelings of warmth and rapid reddening of neck, chest and face.
- Soft tissue - Tendons, ligaments, skin, fat, muscles, nerves and blood vessels.
- Syncope - Fainting or loss of consciousness.
- Tethered Cord Syndrome - A neurological disorder caused by tissue attachments to the spinal cord, limiting movement.
- Thoracic - Relating to the upper and middle portion of the spine.
- Thoracic outlet syndrome (TOS) - TOS is a term used to describe a group of disorders that occur when there is compression, injury, or irritation of the nerves and/or blood vessels (arteries and veins) in the lower neck and upper chest area. Thoracic outlet syndrome is named for the space (the thoracic outlet) between your lower neck and upper chest where this grouping of nerves and blood vessels is found. [6]
- Uterine - Of or relating to the uterus.
- Urticaria - A skin rash triggered by a reaction to food, medicine or other irritants.

[1] "Idiopathic Intracranial Hypertension." *National Eye Institute (NEI)*. NEI Office of Science Communication, April 2014. Web. 2 September 2017.

[2] Zaqqa M, Massumi A. Neurally Mediated Syncope. Texas Heart Institute Journal. 2000;27(3):268-272.

[3] Freeman R, Wieling W, Axelrod FB, et al. Consensus statement on the definition of orthostatic hypotension, neurally mediated syncope and the postural tachycardia syndrome. Clin Auton Res. 2011;21(2):69–72

[4] Low PA, Opfer-Gehrking TL, McPhee BR, et al. . Prospective evaluation of clinical characteristics of orthostatic hypotension. Mayo Clin Proc. 1995;70(7):617–622

[5] Stewart JM. Common Syndromes of Orthostatic Intolerance. Pediatrics. 2013;131(5):968-980. doi:10.1542/peds.2012-2610.

[6] "Thoracic Outlet Syndrome (TOS)." *Cleveland Clinic*. Cleveland Clinic. Web. 2 September 2017.

If you suspect you may have any of the Ehlers-Danlos syndromes, read the most recent, published, international findings, and speak with a physician to go over your concerns. This journal can even be used in preparation for your initial appointment and might provide helpful information for any interested specialists.

If you are not already officially diagnosed with any of the Ehlers-Danlos Syndromes, or any other disease that requires specified logging of activities, please consult with a licensed medical physician of your choosing. This is not intended to be any form of medical diagnostic material. As of March of 2017, the most recent publishing of relevant information was March, 15 2017. A work published by the American Journal of Medical Genetics, Seminars in Medical Genetics, Part C., which consisted of 246 pages of 17 research articles and reviews, including the 2017 International Consortium on the Ehlers-Danlos syndromes.

Thank you for journaling your
Every Day Simple Needs.

THANK YOU

I hope this has been a much-needed tool for you to organize your symptoms and ailments, and propel you into a healthier connection with yourself and others.

This journal is in no way intended to diagnose, or treat the Ehlers-Danlos syndromes, or any other condition. This is a tool to aid those living with chronic and sometimes debilitating disorders.

If you think you have any chronic condition, any of the Ehlers-Danlos syndromes, or any other symptom of concern, please seek medical attention and advice.

Your mindset is the most powerful tool you wield.

2019

JANUARY
S	M	T	W	T	F	S
		1	2	3	4	5
6	7	8	9	10	11	12
13	14	15	16	17	18	19
20	21	22	23	24	25	26
27	28	29	30	31		

FEBRUARY
S	M	T	W	T	F	S
					1	2
3	4	5	6	7	8	9
10	11	12	13	14	15	16
17	18	19	20	21	22	23
24	25	26	27	28		

MARCH
S	M	T	W	T	F	S
					1	2
3	4	5	6	7	8	9
10	11	12	13	14	15	16
17	18	19	20	21	22	23
24	25	26	27	28	29	30
31						

APRIL
S	M	T	W	T	F	S
	1	2	3	4	5	6
7	8	9	10	11	12	13
14	15	16	17	18	19	20
21	22	23	24	25	26	27
28	29	30				

MAY
S	M	T	W	T	F	S
			1	2	3	4
5	6	7	8	9	10	11
12	13	14	15	16	17	18
19	20	21	22	23	24	25
26	27	28	29	30	31	

JUNE
S	M	T	W	T	F	S
						1
2	3	4	5	6	7	8
9	10	11	12	13	14	15
16	17	18	19	20	21	22
23	24	25	26	27	28	29
30						

JULY
S	M	T	W	T	F	S
	1	2	3	4	5	6
7	8	9	10	11	12	13
14	15	16	17	18	19	20
21	22	23	24	25	26	27
28	29	30	31			

AUGUST
S	M	T	W	T	F	S
				1	2	3
4	5	6	7	8	9	10
11	12	13	14	15	16	17
18	19	20	21	22	23	24
25	26	27	28	29	30	31

SEPTEMBER
S	M	T	W	T	F	S
1	2	3	4	5	6	7
8	9	10	11	12	13	14
15	16	17	18	19	20	21
22	23	24	25	26	27	28
29	30					

OCTOBER
S	M	T	W	T	F	S
		1	2	3	4	5
6	7	8	9	10	11	12
13	14	15	16	17	18	19
20	21	22	23	24	25	26
27	28	29	30	31		

NOVEMBER
S	M	T	W	T	F	S
					1	2
3	4	5	6	7	8	9
10	11	12	13	14	15	16
17	18	19	20	21	22	23
24	25	26	27	28	29	30

DECEMBER
S	M	T	W	T	F	S
1	2	3	4	5	6	7
8	9	10	11	12	13	14
15	16	17	18	19	20	21
22	23	24	25	26	27	28
29	30	31				

2020

JANUARY
S	M	T	W	T	F	S
			1	2	3	4
5	6	7	8	9	10	11
12	13	14	15	16	17	18
19	20	21	22	23	24	25
26	27	28	29	30	31	

FEBRUARY
S	M	T	W	T	F	S
						1
2	3	4	5	6	7	8
9	10	11	12	13	14	15
16	17	18	19	20	21	22
23	24	25	26	27	28	29

MARCH
S	M	T	W	T	F	S
1	2	3	4	5	6	7
8	9	10	11	12	13	14
15	16	17	18	19	20	21
22	23	24	25	26	27	28
29	30	31				

APRIL
S	M	T	W	T	F	S
			1	2	3	4
5	6	7	8	9	10	11
12	13	14	15	16	17	18
19	20	21	22	23	24	25
26	27	28	29	30		

MAY
S	M	T	W	T	F	S
					1	2
3	4	5	6	7	8	9
10	11	12	13	14	15	16
17	18	19	20	21	22	23
24	25	26	27	28	29	30
31						

JUNE
S	M	T	W	T	F	S
	1	2	3	4	5	6
7	8	9	10	11	12	13
14	15	16	17	18	19	20
21	22	23	24	25	26	27
28	29	30				

JULY
S	M	T	W	T	F	S
			1	2	3	4
5	6	7	8	9	10	11
12	13	14	15	16	17	18
19	20	21	22	23	24	25
26	27	28	29	30	31	

AUGUST
S	M	T	W	T	F	S
						1
2	3	4	5	6	7	8
9	10	11	12	13	14	15
16	17	18	19	20	21	22
23	24	25	26	27	28	29
30	31					

SEPTEMBER
S	M	T	W	T	F	S
		1	2	3	4	5
6	7	8	9	10	11	12
13	14	15	16	17	18	19
20	21	22	23	24	25	26
27	28	29	30			

OCTOBER
S	M	T	W	T	F	S
				1	2	3
4	5	6	7	8	9	10
11	12	13	14	15	16	17
18	19	20	21	22	23	24
25	26	27	28	29	30	31

NOVEMBER
S	M	T	W	T	F	S
1	2	3	4	5	6	7
8	9	10	11	12	13	14
15	16	17	18	19	20	21
22	23	24	25	26	27	28
29	30	31				

DECEMBER
S	M	T	W	T	F	S
		1	2	3	4	5
6	7	8	9	10	11	12
13	14	15	16	17	18	19
20	21	22	23	24	25	26
27	28	29	30	31		

2021

JANUARY
S	M	T	W	T	F	S
					1	2
3	4	5	6	7	8	9
10	11	12	13	14	15	16
17	18	19	20	21	22	23
24	25	26	27	28	29	30
31						

FEBRUARY
S	M	T	W	T	F	S
	1	2	3	4	5	6
7	8	9	10	11	12	13
14	15	16	17	18	19	20
21	22	23	24	25	26	27
28						

MARCH
S	M	T	W	T	F	S
	1	2	3	4	5	6
7	8	9	10	11	12	13
14	15	16	17	18	19	20
21	22	23	24	25	26	27
28	29	30	31			

APRIL
S	M	T	W	T	F	S
				1	2	3
4	5	6	7	8	9	10
11	12	13	14	15	16	17
18	19	20	21	22	23	24
25	26	27	28	29	30	

MAY
S	M	T	W	T	F	S
						1
2	3	4	5	6	7	8
9	10	11	12	13	14	15
16	17	18	19	20	21	22
23	24	25	26	27	28	29
30	31					

JUNE
S	M	T	W	T	F	S
		1	2	3	4	5
6	7	8	9	10	11	12
13	14	15	16	17	18	19
20	21	22	23	24	25	26
27	28	29	30			

JULY
S	M	T	W	T	F	S
				1	2	3
4	5	6	7	8	9	10
11	12	13	14	15	16	17
18	19	20	21	22	23	24
25	26	27	28	29	30	31

AUGUST
S	M	T	W	T	F	S
1	2	3	4	5	6	7
8	9	10	11	12	13	14
15	16	17	18	19	20	21
22	23	24	25	26	27	28
29	30	31				

SEPTEMBER
S	M	T	W	T	F	S
			1	2	3	4
5	6	7	8	9	10	11
12	13	14	15	16	17	18
19	20	21	22	23	24	25
26	27	28	29	30		

OCTOBER
S	M	T	W	T	F	S
					1	2
3	4	5	6	7	8	9
10	11	12	13	14	15	16
17	18	19	20	21	22	23
24	25	26	27	28	29	30
31						

NOVEMBER
S	M	T	W	T	F	S
	1	2	3	4	5	6
7	8	9	10	11	12	13
14	15	16	17	18	19	20
21	22	23	24	25	26	27
28	29	30				

DECEMBER
S	M	T	W	T	F	S
			1	2	3	4
5	6	7	8	9	10	11
12	13	14	15	16	17	18
19	20	21	22	23	24	25
26	27	28	29	30	31	

2022

JANUARY
S	M	T	W	T	F	S
						1
2	3	4	5	6	7	8
9	10	11	12	13	14	15
16	17	18	19	20	21	22
23	24	25	26	27	28	29
30	31					

FEBRUARY
S	M	T	W	T	F	S
		1	2	3	4	5
6	7	8	9	10	12	13
13	14	15	16	17	18	19
20	21	22	23	24	25	26
27	28					

MARCH
S	M	T	W	T	F	S
		1	2	3	4	5
6	7	8	9	10	11	12
13	14	15	16	17	18	19
20	21	22	23	24	25	26
27	28	29	30	31		

APRIL
S	M	T	W	T	F	S
					1	2
3	4	5	6	7	8	9
10	11	12	13	14	15	16
17	18	19	20	21	22	23
24	25	26	27	28	29	30

MAY
S	M	T	W	T	F	S
1	2	3	4	5	6	7
8	9	10	11	12	13	14
15	16	17	18	19	20	21
22	23	24	25	26	27	28
29	30	31				

JUNE
S	M	T	W	T	F	S
			1	2	3	4
5	6	7	8	9	10	11
12	13	14	15	16	17	18
19	20	21	22	23	24	25
26	27	28	29	30		

JULY
S	M	T	W	T	F	S
					1	2
3	4	5	6	7	8	9
10	11	12	13	14	15	16
17	18	19	20	21	22	23
24	25	26	27	28	29	30
31						

AUGUST
S	M	T	W	T	F	S
	1	2	3	4	5	6
7	8	9	10	11	12	13
14	15	16	17	18	19	20
21	22	23	24	25	26	27
28	29	30	31			

SEPTEMBER
S	M	T	W	T	F	S
				1	2	3
4	5	6	7	8	9	10
11	12	13	14	15	16	17
18	19	20	21	22	23	24
25	26	27	28	29	30	

OCTOBER
S	M	T	W	T	F	S
						1
2	3	4	5	6	7	8
9	10	11	12	13	14	15
16	17	18	19	20	21	22
23	24	25	26	27	28	29
30	31					

NOVEMBER
S	M	T	W	T	F	S
		1	2	3	4	5
6	7	8	9	10	11	12
13	14	15	16	17	18	19
20	21	22	23	24	25	26
27	28	29	30			

DECEMBER
S	M	T	W	T	F	S
				1	2	3
4	5	6	7	8	9	10
11	12	13	14	15	16	17
18	19	20	21	22	23	24
25	26	27	28	29	30	31

www.ingramcontent.com/pod-product-compliance
Lightning Source LLC
Chambersburg PA
CBHW070138210526
45170CB00014B/1455